SURVIVING

KIDNEY DISEASE

True Stories of Love, Courage, Hope, and Heroism

...and a Roadmap for Prevention

FOR MORE INFORMATION, PLEASE VISIT:

www.MichaelFisherMD.com

SURVIVING

KIDNEY DISEASE

True Stories of Love, Courage, Hope, and Heroism

...and a Roadmap for Prevention

Con Capítulos Críticos en Español

MICHAEL B. FISHER MD

Editor: Mick Kronman
Cover Art: Nancy Greenberg
Interior Design: Bonnie Landau
Publisher: Fisher and Allyn MD Inc.

ISBN-10: 0-692-10024-5
ISBN-13: 978-0-692-10024-0

First Edition
Printed in the USA

www.MichaelFisherMD.com

For my patients

Table of Contents

Acknowledgements

Like links in a chain, each solid and solitary yet inextricably connected to links prior and following, such is the nature of acknowledgments presented here. From the first link to the last, they connect waypoints of a life that led me to write this book. From childhood wonder to revelations ensuing from my own lung-cancer surgery, they are parts of the same whole, nothing separating them but time and place.

It started with a compassionate, loving mom who fought for the underserved before it was vogue, and a kind dad who loved children. He was also a coach, whose motivational style I inherited. He taught challenged kids as well as "normal" ones—not so common in the 1950s. My parents set my course and gave me confidence and vision, for which they deserve eternal credit.

In school, the chain of gratitude began with Ruth Kutick, my 6th grade teacher, who wrote in my yearbook, "Someday I will be proud to say he was one of my boys." She made me feel special, and challenged me to do my best. I will always remember her smiling face.

Dr. Phil Stein, my organic-chemistry professor at Brooklyn College, understood my passion to attend medical school. He encouraged me to work hard and compartmentalize tasks to logically and efficiently approach challenges—guidance I follow to this day.

At State University Medical School in Syracuse, pathology professor Dr. David Jones's pioneering work on the anatomy and physiology of the glomerulus inspired me to focus on nephrology. Dr. David Snyder made my nephrology rotation during internship fascinating and exciting. Examining urine under a microscope, the "poor man's kidney biopsy," rendered esoteric diagnoses from just a single drop. After working with Dr. Snyder, I fully committed to pursuing a career in nephrology, a decision I have never regretted.

During my residency and fellowship at UCLA, several doctors profoundly influenced me with their knowledge, expertise and diagnostic acumen.

Dr. David Lee, attending nephrologist at UCLA with whom I made rounds, was a superb physician and a world-class instructor whose seminars to fellows inspired and educated far beyond the norm. Dr. Leslie Dornfeld, rheumatologist and nephrologist, helped make immunologic renal diseases more understandable, especially as new research data emerged. He introduced me to UCLA's Lupus Clinic, where I began to better understand pathological relationships between autoimmune disorders and kidney disease.

Dr. Harvey Gonick may have been my most influential mentor at UCLA. He took me under his wing and taught me how to think critically about medical problems, from heavy-metal poisoning to varied forms of renal dysfunction. He taught me the complex mechanisms of kidney disease, sometimes following 6:00 am tennis matches. He also urged me to enter practice, and we became colleagues soon after. Many times, I referred complex cases to him for his analysis and expertise.

Dr. Thomas Allyn, friend and partner in our Santa Barbara nephrology practice, has been a constant reminder to always pursue excellence in any endeavor. How fortunate for me to have witnessed and shared his excellence and expertise for 37 years.

Drs. Darol Joseph, David Donor and Bindu Kamal, extraordinary nephrologists, have, through their excellence, contributed mightily to my professional growth and development.

Dr. Louis Rubin and his wife Ruth, among our oldest friends, arrived in Santa Barbara in 1975, two months after we arrived. Their support during my illnesses was strong. Dr. Rubin, a highly skilled Urologist, assisted in my surgery for diverticulitis and helped save my life. Leslie and I are so grateful for their friendship.

To clinical staff, who treat acutely ill hospital patients or work each day with renewed commitment to compassion and medical excellence in our dialysis unit, I offer my deepest appreciation. They do the heavy lifting upon which my practice and our patients depend. Martha Hilken, Mondra Randal, Suzie Gosnell and Amy Qadri perform magnificently with sick patients requiring emergency dialysis. Florna Delarmente, Director of Nursing at the Santa Barbara Artificial Kidney Center, will always have my admiration for making the Center a beacon of excellence. Fernando Mendoza, our clinical Physician Assistant, has skillfully attended to patients' emotional and medical needs since the Center's inception. He also translated five chapters of this book into Spanish.

Office manager Fern Halperin, put simply, taught me how to run a medical practice. Compassionate and madly efficient, she devoted herself to our practice for over three decades, greeting patients and chatting with them as they awaited me in sterile, emotionless exam rooms. Trained in nursing, she also gave silky-smooth injections. Fern was family to me and my wife Leslie, and like an older sister to our three kids.

Elizabeth McWhirter succeeded Fern, and to this day provides the same, top-notch personalized care. She is beloved by all who know her. I'm also indebted to professionals who work outside our offices and clinic, whose excellence in the field and commitment to extending life and enhancing quality of life for kidney patients deserve recognition. There are many to thank, but I especially wish to recognize doctors and nurses at Cedars Sinai Medical Center, our partners in renal immunology and transplantation.

Dr. Stanley Jordan, Cedars' Director of Kidney Transplantation and Transplant Immunology, has helped initiate breakthroughs that allow successful transplants for "sensitized" patients who've had previous transplants and need another, as well as non-blood-type-compatible transplants. Dr. Jordan has helped save and extend countless lives.

Dr. Louis Cohen, surgical director of Cedars' kidney transplant program, has transplanted thousands of kidneys, many the second, third, even fourth for the same patient, adroitly managing myriad surgical challenges along the way. His wisdom, commitment, and service to the transplant community have been nothing short of monumental.

Several non-medical professionals also made valuable contributions to this book, beginning with my wife of 47 years, Leslie Fisher, whose love and support through good times and bad I will forever cherish. An editor in her own right, Leslie read and reread every chapter. Her keen observations and suggestions helped immensely. My friend and Iyengar Yoga mentor, Richard McLaughlin, whose support after my lung surgery was invaluable. His patience, compassion and expertise in the yoga studio accelerated my healing.

I offer thanks, also, to people who helped bring this book to life. Linda Cashdan of The Word Process, author and book doctor, helped me organize my thoughts with careful editing, while teaching me how to publish a book. Mick Kronman, a published author and case-study in this book, applied his writing and editing skills to help capture the power and inspiration of patients' stories. Author Michael Bowker helped get an initial manuscript of this book in the hands of a New York City literary agent. His professional skills were invaluable. I thank him for that. I am grateful to Dorothy Sewell, my patient and friend, for her acute last-minute editing. My wonderful wife Leslie, who was an editor of her school newspaper, and Mick's wife Ginger, one of the heroes in this book, both took out the magnifying glass and scrupulously found nagging errors in the manuscript, which they corrected. I owe thanks, also, to Lucinda Rae, who photographed me and contributed to the book's cover design.

Finally, a word about patients profiled in this book, patients I've had the honor and privilege of serving. They taught me life-lessons I could learn no other way, lessons of love, fortitude, patience, perseverance, courage and hope. They taught me that when these attributes alloy, near-inconceivable results are possible.

They are my heroes and the heroes of this book.

Introduction

If you are reading this, there's a good chance you, a loved one, friend, colleague, or acquaintance have been diagnosed with kidney disease. Nearly 30 million Americans—almost 10%—suffer kidney ailments, yet a diagnosis can make you feel terribly alone, cut off from the world and your prior life. It's as if you've suddenly plunged down the proverbial Rabbit Hole, into a new existence filled with procedures, diagnoses, doctors, tests and long medical terms you've never heard. It can be frightening, confusing, isolating.

Initially, I wrote this book to honor my most challenged and challenging patients whose courage and success overcoming the kidney-failure nightmare guided me through my own challenge with cancer. Their true sagas urge, even implore, you to maintain hope, and let you know you are not alone. Many of us do care about you and there are answers to the multitude of questions you may have.

Most important, there are plenty of great reasons to believe you can enjoy a long, fulfilling life, even with an advanced diagnosis. Proof lies in the inspiring stories from my own patients, who, in their own words, describe how they overcame astonishing physical and psychological challenges and now live rich, meaningful lives. They provide moving, often amazing, evidence of how high the human spirit can soar. Truth, indeed, is stranger than fiction, as you will see in the pages ahead.

This book is also highly practical, providing information that will arm you with knowledge to control your situation, whether you're a patient, caregiver, loved one, or friend.

As a doctor and kidney specialist, and part of the University of

Southern California School of Medicine for the past 35 years, I have treated thousands of patients suffering from a variety of kidney ailments. During this time, I've searched for books that would help my patients not only understand their disease by explaining pathologies in layman's language, but explain the complex and serious psychological and emotional challenges they face. When I couldn't find a book that covered both topics, each critical for patient care, I decided to write it myself. This is the result, and I hope it provides hope and guidance for patients to find their own path back to good health.

I have included a primer to kidney diseases, which explains how kidneys function, what happens when they fail, and available treatments. It addresses the Spartan restrictions in diet, fluid intake, and lifestyle changes necessary for survival. Hopefully, it motivates dialysis patients and provides them the tools needed to adhere to and comply with a difficult, prescriptive regimen so they can reach the goal of a successful kidney transplant.

Other chapters include a look at future treatments, including the exciting development of a bio-mechanical kidney, prevention and wellness, renal transplantation, and a detailed look at steps necessary to get that transplant. Much of the second half of the book is to provide knowledge, based on experience and science, to empower each reader to utilize the suggestions, and to seize the tools to prevent the serious diseases now in epidemic proportion that are so commonplace. I speak of obesity, diabetes, kidney failure, heart disease, hypertension and cancer.

The book also explores the all-important relationship between you and your doctor. I know the critical nature of that relationship, not only from my own practice, but because for the past few years my role has been reversed—I became the patient when diagnosed with serious lung cancer in 2013. After being on one end of the spectrum as a doctor for more than three decades, I suddenly found myself on what I call the "medical conveyor belt," where you feel as if you've lost control over your own life, moved from test to test, procedure to procedure, in an often-impersonal, cold, frightening, system. It can overwhelm and confuse, sometimes leaving you feeling more like a number than a human being.

I understand what you may be going through because I've gone through it. That experience, more than anything else, motivated me to write this book, which endeavors, among other things, to explain ways to stop the conveyor belt and gain the personalized treatment you deserve.

This book is also about regaining health – your health. I wrote it to help you and people who care about you understand and successfully address kidney disease, and to help provide hope and conviction that you can face whatever challenges lie ahead. You can return to an exciting, productive, healthy life. I've seen it happen a thousand times. You are not alone. We are all in this together.

Writing the manuscript for this book, I realized many patients I wrote about had early-life, emotional trauma that resulted in what I consider severe chronic stress. Their illnesses manifested during this time and ultimately lead to kidney failure. Observations over the course of my 50-year practice strongly suggested that in many patients a pattern of organic disease following a period of chronic stress. Writing this book allowed me the opportunity to study the relatively new sciences of psychoneuroimmunology and epigenetics to see if compelling, documented evidence of this relationship exists. It does.

Genetic makeup, of course, is an overwhelming factor determining what sicknesses we will acquire during our lifetime. I agree, however, with Dr. William Osler, the father of modern medicine, who, in the first edition of his textbook of medicine in 1892, discussed the etiology (cause) of what was likely rheumatoid arthritis, which he called arthritis deformans. "It is difficult to separate some cases from ordinary chronic rheumatism, but the multiple form has, in all probability, a nervous origin," he wrote. His view was based on facts like a strong association of the disease with shock, worry, and grief, concluding this was not coincidence.

I'm convinced that if we can develop a deeper understanding of ourselves and are willing to modify a potentially toxic environment that envelops each of us daily, we can overcome high stress, poor nutrition, sedentary behavior, and the diminishing role of family and friends in our lives. Worldwide, people who live the longest, embrace this simple formula, this principle, as life's core value.

Even though the vignettes that you will read are about people who overcame a variety of kidney ailments that at the time appeared insurmountable, their collective stories provide a metaphor for the strength of the human spirit. Never forget: you're stronger than you think, and you'll prove it when faced with unexpected calamity, be it cancer, loss of a spouse or child, divorce, foreclosure, bankruptcy, hurricane, wildfire, or kidney disease. Your resilience isn't fixed or finite. In the cradle of hope, love, knowledge, and determination, you can overcome far more than you may believe possible.

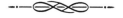

Chapter 1

Michael

In 2013, I faced minor surgery to remove a small mass on my tongue. It was biopsied in Santa Barbara, with non-definitive results—likely either an infection or cancer. Could my years-long exposure to powerful drugs that block a protein called tumor necrosis factor alpha, an important component of the immune system, relate to my tongue problem? Was it a consequence of, or a tradeoff for, the positive effects of these medicines on a chronic illness I had? Did it result from long-term immunosuppression?

Protocol at the UCLA Medical Center required I get a chest x-ray in preparation for surgical removal of the mass in my tongue. I wasn't happy about it and balked at having another x-ray. I was a non-smoker and I'd had a chest film only two years prior, results of which were perfectly normal. In the end, however, I decided to be a good patient and do it.

I didn't think much more about the x-ray until a radiologist and I reviewed the film, where we could clearly see a density in my upper left lung. My jaw dropped, my heart raced, and an existential clamminess flushed through me from head to toe.

Although the differential diagnosis for my tongue was between an infection and cancer, without question, in my mind, cancer was now much more likely. (Thankfully, it was an infection and successfully treated.)

That's when everything turned on its head. With an odd combination of professional respect, compassion, and objectivity, the radiologist spoke to me the same way he'd discussed my patients when analyzing *their* films. I tried to engage him dispassionately, but I couldn't stem a powerful, foreboding sense of danger spreading over me. I was no longer just a physician, no longer part of the "temporarily healthy." In one terrifying moment, I channeled the anxiety I'd seen in my patients' eyes during the preceding 40 years.

I was now one of them.

After a CT scan confirmed what the x-ray showed, a team of physicians examined me, developed an action plan, and processed me into the medical machinery. It felt robotic, like queuing up to enter some parallel dimension, but I knew even then I was lucky to be in great hands and in the "action mode" so swiftly.

My oncologist, Dr. Alan Rosenblum, was frank and dutiful, yet compassionate and hopeful. His brilliance inspired trust. Still, I felt control slip away as I rode the medical conveyer belt from test to test, procedure to procedure, culminating in surgery to remove the upper lobe of my left lung.

The next time I thought about my kidney patients I was lying on a cold, stone-hard procedure table in the radiology suite awaiting a lung biopsy, results of which would decide my fate. Waiting quietly and alone for the radiologist to enter the room, I recalled countless times I had discussed kidney biopsies with patients whose life-altering diagnoses depended on somebody peering at tiny cells through a microscope. If I recommend a renal biopsy in the future, I told myself, counting dots on acoustic ceiling tiles above me, I would better educate and better prepare the patient over time.

Dr. Arthur Lee, an expert in invasive radiology, good friend, and colleague, entered the room, thankfully interrupting my descent into self-analysis. Dr. Lee explained that the mass in my lung was near large blood vessels, and if he used a large-bore needle, bleeding could result. Dr. Lee told me there was a better chance of obtaining tissue with the larger needle, but if he couldn't obtain tissue using a safer, smaller needle, I would need surgery to get a satisfactory sample.

A tradeoff loomed. I include this here because so often treating kidney disease, patients face serious decisions that come as a sobering surprise. You think doctors know the best way to handle everything, yet they may well ask you to help make medical decisions that could alter your life.

I recommend that you prepare yourself for this, and don't let it confuse or depress you. There are ways to gather information, so your decision is wise and well-considered. Again, this is where the trusting bond with your doctor is paramount. You need to respect his or her consulting advice and listen to it before making your own decision. Your support network—family, friends, and others—become important consultants during this time as well, but your doctor should always be your lead consultant.

I had tremendous confidence in Dr. Lee's technical ability, so we chose the riskier path, the larger needle. As he explained its potential complications, I again recalled warning my patients of possible severe bleeding, the potential need for emergency surgery, even the possibility of death from a kidney biopsy. I felt what most of them must feel—uncertainty and fear.

As time passed, I felt more and more like a character in a Franz Kafka novel who wakes up each morning, feeling fine, then one morning, he looks in the mirror and sees himself dressed in hospital garb. I heard myself, in a raspy voice, whispering, "Your role as a physician is over. You're a patient now, with not just any illness, but life-threatening lung cancer." I'm sure my own patients, many of whom learned of their disease during routine physical exams, have felt the same.

The biopsy left me physically sore, but nothing compared to the mental anguish of awaiting its results. During this time, I was keenly aware of seeing life through my patients' eyes. I tried hard to learn everything I could about the experience, even though at times it was hard to gain perspective because facing a serious illness is such a personal, emotional rollercoaster. Still, trying to use the experience to make me a better doctor afforded me a tiny window of detachment.

I recalled one patient, who described seeing lab results curl out of his workplace fax machine: "It has always scared me," he said, "living in limbo, wondering if the results would say I could live carefree for a while or whether I was doomed to another round of biopsies, dialysis, and transplantation. My heart would pound so hard my visual field pulsed in rhythm as I ripped the results from the machine, not looking at them until I got inside my office and closed the door, where I could privately indulge my anxieties. Then I would arrange the paper in such a manner that I could use a ruler and go line by line, seeing what each result indicated, too scared to see the 'whole' of the results at once. It was stupid, but that's the only way I could handle it."

I told him I didn't think it stupid at all. In fact, I considered it a wise strategy that both protected his emotions and allowed him to better understand the results. I recommend these kinds of mini-strategies to my patients, to devise their own stress-relieving methods for dealing with test results and other anxiety-inducing parts of a journey of many medical miles. Even today, three and a half years post-surgery and still on medicine, a frightful twitch rattles me awaiting scan results.

My oncologist and I hoped for the best, feared the worst, and expected something in between. That's what we got. Biopsy results and lung scans suggested the mass was malignant and included a local lymph node, but hadn't spread further, I felt optimistic that removing one lobe of my lung would excise it. Combined with chemotherapy (a new "designer drug" specific for this cancer), I felt I stood a good chance of beating this thing. He even said I probably wouldn't lose my hair. This gave me a huge sense of relief, a little odd considering what else was at stake. Still, I had optimism and hope, vitally important to overcoming maladies of every stripe.

The Precious Gift of Time

The surgery was successful, but with notable complications. I had been placed on my right side with much weight on my right hip, so the surgeon could work on my left lung at the proper orientation to remove the malignancy. As a result, the operation hampered my walking for months due to resultant bursitis in the affected hip. In addition, as the left lung began to take over space in the left chest cavity, a kink developed in the large bronchus, or airway tube, that provides air to the left lung. This left me with considerable shortness of breath plus an ominous wheeze when I drew a big breath.

Recovery, therefore, was difficult and brought with it another set of physical and emotional challenges. One of these, faced by so many patients with serious illnesses, was determining how much to interact with the "world outside" while on the mend. Too much interaction can rob your energy, while not enough can make you feel isolated. I chose to spend time only with family and close friends. Many wonderful people inquired about my health, but I didn't emerge from my protective shell until I got past excessive weakness that accompanies the process, plus enough "clear" scans to buoy my confidence and optimism. I began practicing more yoga and worked with my Iyengar yoga teacher to gain strength and improve my pulmonary function, utilizing an ancient breathing technique called pranayama.

I'm well again now, gaining strength, able to see patients, and live a more normal, active life. One patient even told me recently, "Seeing you with a spring in your step gives me great joy," which in turn made *me* feel great joy. My tumor remains undetectable.

I realize now, more than ever, that time is a precious gift. Thomas Mann, the German novelist and philosopher, was once asked what he valued most in life. "The transitory nature of life," he said. "But is not transitoriness—the perishableness of life—something very sad? No! It is the very soul of existence. It imparts value, dignity, interest, to life. Transitoriness creates time, and time is the essence."

Time gives us an opportunity to accumulate self-knowledge, grow as individuals, accomplish goals and find meaning in life. Making sound decisions is critical to maximizing that time. If I had stubbornly refused that chest x-ray, arguing that I'd just had one two years prior, and it was normal, I'm certain they would have gone ahead with the minor surgery. My lung cancer would have spread, and likely I would not be sharing these thoughts with you now. A cliché is a cliché only because it's true, and surely, "A Physician who treats himself has a fool for a patient."

During my convalescence, I had ample time to reflect on how I could be of additional value to my patients, now that I had walked in their shoes. In that regard, I began to see my battle with cancer as a blessing.

Reviewing my patients' odysseys, from the onset of kidney disease to chronic renal insufficiency and its crippling effects, to those who ultimately received life-restoring kidney transplants, I began to fully understand the power of the human spirit and will to live. Many of my patients summoned the noblest of human qualities—courage, resilience, determination, and hope—to overcome their complex illnesses. Their attitudes and actions inspired me during my own months of uncertainty and recovery, and I was driven to share their compelling stories.

I thought about family members and friends who came forward without hesitation to give the "gift of life"—one of their kidneys—to save people they love. I recalled the early days of kidney transplantation, in the 1960s and 1970s, when nobody knew the long-term consequence of living with only one kidney. Still, mothers, fathers, sisters, and brothers selflessly and heroically donated, risking their lives for family members. Simply put, real heroes don't throw touchdown passes or hit home runs. They donate kidneys.

We've learned over the past 35 years, of course, that if a donor is meticulously screened and in good health, they'll likely live a normal life—great news since demand for donor kidneys continues escalating as kidney disease skyrockets worldwide, closely linked to a global epidemic of diabetes. Much has been written about this, but even textbooks on the subject lack a certain pathos or explanation about the galactic emotional effects renal disease can have on patients, loved ones and transplant donors. Hopefully, through stories like ones in this book, we can stand together and successfully wage war on kidney disease and its causes.

In William Ernest Henley's poem *Invictus,* the author has lost a limb to tuberculosis and is in danger of losing his remaining leg and likely his life. Still, he maintains inner strength and courage. The poem was a favorite of former South African President Nelson Mandela, who spent 27 years in prison and often encouraged others by reciting it. The movie *Invictus*, set in South Africa, also addressed issues of meeting human struggle with internal courage.

Invictus

Out of the night that covers me
Black as the pit from pole to pole,
I thank whatever gods may be
For my unconquerable soul.

In the fell clutch of circumstance
I have not winced nor cried aloud,
Under the bludgeoning of chance
My head is bloody, but unbowed.

Beyond this place of wrath and tears
Looms but the Horror of the shade,
And yet the menace of the years,
Finds and shall find me unafraid.

It matters not how straight the gait,
How charged with punishment the scroll,
I am the master of my fate,
I am the captain of my soul.

For kidney patients, I hope you similarly refuse to give up the battle for life, and continue, in any manner possible, pursuing transplantation. The stories of my patients, though diverse in personalities, circumstances, and types of kidney disease—and decisively uncommon for their life–imitates-art twists and turns—reflect what can be achieved amid the most daunting, life-threatening circumstances.

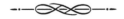

Capítulo 1

Michael

El protocolo de UCLA Medical Center indicaba que seria necesario obtener una radiografía de tórax en preparación para la cirugía la semana siguiente. Yo la verdad no creía que fuera necesario tener otra radiografia del pecho. Para que?. Yo me dije: para que? yo no fumo y lo mas que he fumado fue 1 cigarillo como dos años antes, y pensé que los resultados serian perfectamente normales. Pero al final, sin embargo, decidí ser un buen paciente y lo hice. Recuerdo que cuando el radiólogo revisó la imagen, mi mandíbula cayó, mi corazón palpitaba rapidamente, y sentía una rara debilidad existencial que empezaba en mí cabeza y avanzaba hasta los dedos de mis pies. La radiografia mostraba una mancha opaca en la parte superior izquierda de mi pulmon.

Con una extraña combinación de respeto profesional, objetividad y compasión, el radiólogo me habló como si analizara una radiografia de uno de mis pacientes. Lo questione, curioso con el propósito de escuchar su opinión. Pero cuando mencionó la palabra cáncer como parte del diagnóstico, me entro una sensación de premonición de peligro momentáneamente agotando mi capacidad de darse cuenta de lo inevitable: Yo ya no era sólo un médico, ya no era la persona que estaba "temporalmente sano." Este fue un momento terrible. Me entro una sensación de pánico y ansiedad. Algo que nomas solia había visto en los ojos de mis propios pacientes por más de 35 años de mi carrera médica. Ahora yo era el enfermo, yo era uno de ellos.

Al instante, se hizo una tomografía computarizada (CT scan) en ese momento la cual confirmó mi mayor temor, un tumor en mi pulmón. Al instante, un equipo de médicos dirigido por un oncólogo me examinaron, desarrollaron un plan de cuidado y me transforme en material de fabrica. Era un sentimiento robótico, a punto de someterme a una serie de pruebas, estudios y investigaciones como pasando por una banda de fabrica pero tenia la certeza que estaba en buenas manos rodeado de los mejores profesionales médicos y la mejor tecnología listos para vencer este nuevo desafío los mas rápido posible.

Mi especialista de cancer, Dr. Rosenblum, era compasivo, franco, inteligente y un gran motivador. Su sabiduría inspiraba confianza. Pero aún así, sentía que mi vida se descontrolaba y se perdia deslizandoze al ver que mi vida pasaba por una banda médica sometiéndose a prueba tras prueba, procedimiento tras procedimiento, con la meta de extripar el lóbulo superior de mi pulmón.

Se me vino a ala mente mis pacientes. Ahi acostados en una cama dura y fría, como una piedra en la sala de radiología, en espera de una biopsia de pulmón, cuyos resultados decidirían mi destino. Recuerdo, que cuando esperaba al radiólogo entrar a mi cuarto, se me vino a la mente cómo yo solia explicar exactamente lo mismo a mis pacientes de sus biopsias renales. Ahora me doy cuenta el impacto que estos resultados tienen en el resto de sus vidas. Miraba al techo contando los puntitos y pensando como estos resultados cambiarían sus vidas para siempre. Me daba cuenta en este instante como de hoy en adelante, haría lo mejor posible y daría el mayor esfuerzo en educar y preparar a mis pacientes lo mas posible al momento de revelar sus resultados químicos.

Dr. Lee, un buen amigo y colega, entró a mi cuarto, afortunadamente interrumpiendo mi autoanálisis, quien un amigo llama "el peligro de conseguir entrar en su propia cabeza." Después de un intercambio breve y nervioso de trivia, se puso a trabajar seriamente, surrealista, por lo menos. El Dr. Lee explicó que el tumor en mi pulmón estaba muy cerca de vasos sanguíneos, lo cual complicaba su extracción y me explico que al utilizar una aguja de gran diámetro, corria el riesgo de una hemorragia severa. Una preocupaccion alarmente se vislumbraba. Me explico que si usaba un instrumento or abuja mas pequeña q esta quizás no obtendría la muestra deseada y tendría que someterme a otro procedimiento quirúrgico.

Tenía gran confianza en la capacidad medica y técnica del Dr. Lee, así que elegimos el camino más arriesgado, usar la aguja más grande. Al tiempo que me explicaba sus posibles complicaciones, se me vino ala mente como yo advertía a mis pacientes del posible sangrado serio que podía resultar, la necesidad de tener que recurrir a cirugía de emergencia o incluso morir todo por obtener una biopsia de riñón. Sentí lo que mis pacientes sentían, incertidumbre y mucho miedo.

Paso a paso, como si divinamente ordenado, estaba entrando al de mundo de ser paciente. Me sentía como un personaje de una novela de Franz Kafka que se despierta una mañana, se siente bien, entonces mira en el espejo y ve a sí mismo vestido en ropa de hospital, con un susurro de voz ronca, "Tu papel como médico se acabo. Ahora eres un paciente, victima de no cualquier enfermedad pero otra victima de cáncer, una enfermedad fatal que poco a poco te va robando tu vida. Estoy seguro de que mis propios pacientes, muchos de los cuales se enteraron de su enfermedad durante exámenes físicos de rutina, sentían lo mismo.

La biopsia me dejó adolorido, pero nada comparado con la inquietud de la espera de sus resultados. Por ahora, ver mi condición a través de los ojos — mios y los cientos de pacientes que había tratado, era una sensación rara e inescapable. Era parte de mi ADN, no había razón para luchar contra él. Particularmente recuerdo un paciente que describió con gran inquietud ver como los resultados se deslizaban por la maquina de fax del trabajo: Decia " Me asustaba saber y siempre tenia miedo el saber o no saber si vas vivir otro dia mas , si vas a depender de mas pruebas, mas estudios, mas biopsies, dialysis o transplante". Mi corazón palpitaba tan duro que mi campo visual pulsaba tanto al punto que arrancaba los resultados de la máquina de fax, recuerdo no mirarlos hasta que entraba en mi oficina y puerta cerrada, y ya privadamente podía lamentar mis angustias. Recuerdo agarrar una regla y leer renglón por renglón, línea por línea como no queriendo ver el resultado completo.

Esto suena estúpido pero para mi era la mejor manera de asimilar y manejar lo que estaba pasando.

Mi oncólogo y yo esperabamos lo mejor, temíamos lo peor y nos consolábamos con algo positivo de por medio. Y eso es lo que obtuvimos. Resultados de la biopsia y las exploraciones del pulmón sugieren la lesion era, de hecho, mala e incluia una grandula linfatica, pero no se había regado mas de lo esperado y hubo considerable optimismo que extreyendo parte de mi pulmón seria lo mas apropiado. Combinado con quimoterapia (una nueva "medicina de marca" específica para este tipo de cáncer), tuve la certeza de que podía vencer este problema. Dr. Lee estaba tan tranquilo y confidente en su tratamiento que me comento que quizás ni llegaría a perder el pelo a pesar de mis 71 anos de edad. Esto me dio una sensación extraña, inexplicable, de alivio, teniendo en cuenta lo que estaba en juego.

La cirugía fue todo un éxito, sin complicaciones notorias. Mi recuperación, sin embargo trago otro conjunto de desafíos físicos y emocionales.

Tener siempre codiciado mi privacidad, deseaba pasar mas tiempo "libre" (algo que no es suficiente, cualquier médico le dirá) con familia, amigos cercanos y colegas, me encerré en mi propio mundo. Mucha gente maravillosa preguntó acerca de mi salud, pero yo no salía de mi morada hasta que llegué más allá de la debilidad excesiva que acompañaba el estar enfermo. Con mucho autoanálisis mi confianza y optimismo siguió y siguió creciendo. Aún hoy, tres años después de la cirugía y quimioterapia, una sensación espantosa me llena el cuerpo al esperar los resultados del cat scan.

Me siento bien otra vez, cada día recuperando mi fuerza, y hasta capaz de ver a mis pacientes y vivir una nueva vida más normal y activa. Un paciente me dijo recientemente, "Viéndote vivito y coleando me da mucha alegría", que a su vez esto me dio mucho animo y alegría. Mi tumor sigue siendo indetectable. Todas las mañanas, cuando despierto, pienso sobre qué bendición es poder respirar, tener todos mis sentidos, hacer ejercicio, ver a mis pacientes y disfrutar de mi familia y amigos. El tiempo es un regalo precioso, y de alguna manera, siento como que mi tiempo en esta tierra se ha extendido.

Thomas Mann, novelista alemán y filósofo, una vez se le preguntó lo que él valoraba más en la vida. "La corta naturaleza de la vida", dijo. ¿"Pero su longevidad, la perishableness de la vida, algo muy triste? ¡No! Es el alma de la existencia. Imparte valor, dignidad, intereses, a la vida. La corta estancia crea tiempo y tiempo es la esencia de la vida".

El tiempo nos da la oportunidad de adquirir más conocimiento, ideas, crecer como personas, lograr metas y encontrar mayor significado en la vida. Utilizando el tiempo eficazmente, uno puede transformar y alcanzar paz y tranquilidad. Si obstinadamente no me hubiera hecho la radiografía del pecho, y pensando que todo estaba normal, estoy seguro que habría seguido adelante con la cirugía menor que se había planeado. El cáncer se hubiera regado o diseminado, y probablemente yo no estaría escribiendo este libro. Un cliché es un cliche solo porque es cierto, y sin duda, "un médico que se trata de curar a sí mismo es tonto como paciente".

Durante mi convalecencia tuve tiempo suficiente para reflexionar sobre mi vida. Pensé en pacientes con enfermedad renal que he cuidado, como yo, ante una enfermedad mortal. Pensé en cómo ahora yo caminado como paciente en sus zapatos, en una montaña rusa de emociones encontradas.

Repasando casos de mis pacientes, desde el inicio de la enfermedad renal, insuficiencia renal crónica y sus efectos devastadores, a algunas que finalmente recibieron trasplantes de riñón, comienze a entender el poder de la voluntad humana, específicamente el deseo de vivir. Muchos se refugian en las más nobles cualidades humanas, coraje, resistencia, determinación y esperanza — para superar una enfermedad compleja y mortal. Sus historias me motivaron y durante mis meses de incertidumbre y de lenta recuperación y en última instancia inspiraron a que yo escribiera este libro.

Pensé en miembros de la familia y amigos que valientemente sin vacilación se ofrecían para dar el "regalo de vida", uno de sus riñones, para salvar a personas que aman. Recordaba los primeros días del trasplante de riñón, en la década de 1960 y 1970, cuando nadie sabía la consecuencia a largo plazo de vivir con tan sólo un riñón. Aún así, mamas, papas, hermanas, hermanos desinteresadamente y heroicamente ofrecían donar, arriesgando sus vidas para rescatar a los menos afortunados que siendo atados a las máquinas de diálisis por agujas y tubos que al final terminarían con una vida mucho mas corta de lo esperado.

Ahora, aquí está la buena noticia: en los últimos 35 años hemos aprendido que si un donante está meticulosamente seleccionado y de buena salud, tienen una alta probabilidad de vivir una vida normal, esto es algo que anteriormente era una inseguridad.

Mucho se ha escrito sobre la compleja naturaleza de la enfermedad renal, que hasta la fecha sigue alcanzado altas proporciones epidémicas globales con sus efectos catastróficos en los pacientes y sus familias. Aún así, incluso libros de texto sobre el tema carecen de explicaciones acerca de los efectos galácticos que suelen tener en pacientes renales sus familias y donadores.

Recordando historias clínicas de mis pacientes, algunas van más allá de la década de los 70s. Sentí que algunas de sus historias valia la pena contarlas. Si este libro hace más de educar a la gente sobre cómo evitar la enfermedad del riñón, como enfrentar o sobrevivir o donar un riñón a un ser querido, lo considerare un todo un éxito. Si eleva el espíritu de nuevos pacientes diagnosticados (20 millones de americanos sufren algún tipo de enfermedad renal progresiva y se desarrollarán la etapa del extremo enfermedad Renal (ESRD), que, sin diálisis, significa muerte segura), mejor todavía. Si anima a jóvenes nefrólogos y su equipo la salud a un refinado entendimiento global de esta enfermedad y el grande impacto de consecuencias físicas y emocionales que lo acompañan, seria mucho mejor. Si las historias de pacientes sumidos en las arenas movedizas de este problema, y sino fuera por valentía, esperanza y amor extraídas por uno mismo y que puedan vivir vidas normales, incluso extraordinarias, inspiran la emulación, esto seria la mejor meta de todo.

Para la gente que esta pasando por una catástrofe médica, cualquiera sea su causa, las ganas y positividad evidenciado por los pacientes en este libro reflejan una energía incontenible que nunca sucumbe a la oscuridad y la negatividad que disminuyen las posibilidades de supervivencia. Ellos formaron sus destinos, desafiando a los incrédulos o no creyentes (incluso los médicos a veces), y creyendo firmemente en su propia capacidad para forjar un camino de bienestar y buena salud.

Un poema de William Ernest Henley de "Invictus", el autor ha perdido una extremidad a la tuberculosis y corre el riesgo de perder su pierna restante y probablemente su vida. Aún así, mantiene coraje y fuerza interior. Del mismo modo, muchos de mis pacientes se negaron a renunciar a la batalla por la vida y continuaron, de cualquier manera posible, la búsqueda de un trasplante de riñón. Como dice Henley, permanecieron incólumes, confiando en su "alma inconquistable" como "amos de su destino." Mientras encarcelado durante 27 años en la prisión de Robben Island, Nelson Mandela recitada repetidamente "Invictus" a otros presos, levantar sus espíritus y su propia con su mensaje de autodeterminación:

Invictus

De la noche que me cubre
Negro como el hoyo de poste a poste,
Doy gracias a cualesquiera dioses pueden ser
Por mi alma inconquistable.

En el embrague cayó de circunstancia
No he pestañeado ni llorado en voz alta,
Bajo la coacción de oportunidad
Mi cabeza es sangrienta, pero erguida.

Más allá de este lugar de ira y lágrimas
Telares sino el Horror de la sombra,
Y sin embargo, la amenaza de los años,
Encuentra y me encontrará sin miedo.

Es importante no como recto el andar,
Carga con el castigo el rollo,
Yo soy el amo de mi destino,
Yo soy el capitán de mi alma.

Las historias de mis pacientes, aunque diversas en sus personalidades, circunstancias y tipos de enfermedad renal y decididamente poco común para su arte imita la vida de vueltas y revueltas, reflejan lo que puede lograrse en medio de las circunstancias más desalentadoras, peligrosa para la vida.

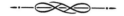

Chapter 2

Kidney Disease, a Primer

As an Associate Clinical Professor of Medicine at the Keck School of Medicine at the University of Southern California, I've taught medical students and residents for decades. They've all told me kidney physiology was one of their most difficult subjects in medical school.

So, hang on while I try to simplify this complicated organ, because understanding the cause, effects, and treatment of kidney disease requires knowing how they work.

With rare exceptions, we're all born with two kidneys. Essentially, they're trash collectors, ridding the body of waste products and toxic substances left over from normal body processes like digestion and muscle activity. Kidneys also maintain normal blood pressure and a normal blood count (the opposite of fatiguing anemia), provide an active form of Vitamin D and protect our bones by maintaining normal bone metabolism.

In this chapter I'll explore how normal kidneys maintain **metabolic balance** (the equilibrium between the intake of nutrients and their eventual loss through absorption or excretion). I'll also explain the critically important role of kidneys as endocrine organs, plus some common diseases that cause kidney failure.

There will be no quiz, but there will be some medical jargon that may be foreign to you. Learning these terms prior to reading patients' stories will, however, enhance understanding of their challenges and victories.

A glossary of medical terms is included at the end of the book, to facilitate a better understanding of renal function and illness, so you can "feel" what kidney patients and organ donors feel.

How Kidneys Work

Each kidney contains about one million microscopic units of function called nephrons (kidney specialists are hence called nephrologists). Each nephron consists of a small blood vessel called an arteriole that delivers blood to even smaller blood vessels called capillaries. They all reside in a structure called a Bowman's Capsule. A space that collects fluid filtered from the blood that has passed through the capillaries separates each capillary from the capsule. A healthy kidney filters blood as it flows through this labyrinth of tiny vessels within Bowman's Capsule. Called the **glomerulus**, it's found in the first segment of the nephron (see figure 1: Diagram of the Nephron). The glomerulus boasts a large surface area to facilitate the filtration process. It allows small particles or molecules to pass through it, while larger particles the body needs remain in the blood, such as blood cells and proteins. In some ways, kidney dialysis simulates this process—extracting toxic stuff and returning the rest. But more on that later.

Blood is forced through the glomerular capillaries at higher pressure than the pressure at which blood generally travels around the body. Assisted by the glomerular capillaries' increased pressure, a filtration process occurs in which normal proteins and cells remain in the blood stream. The blood that is filtered ("filtrate") leaves the glomerulus and moves into a tubular pathway and finally a collecting duct. As fluid moves through the tubules, a spectacular biologic transport system removes waste products while reabsorbing salt, water, and all nutrients essential for metabolic balance. The remaining fluid is urine.

The process and subsequent flow of filtrate through this micro-aq-

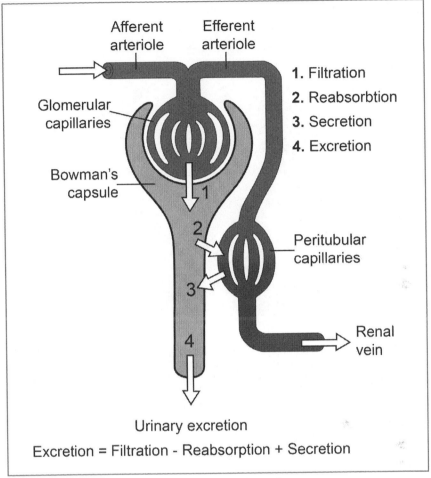

Figure 1: Diagram of the Nephron

ueduct occurs simultaneously in each of the one-million glomeruli in each kidney. Eventually, the filtrate (at this point genuine urine) from each kidney funnels into the collecting ducts, ultimately entering left and right ureters, which pour into the bladder (see figure 2: Diagram of the Kidney System). When the bladder fills with urine, pressure stretches its muscular wall, sending a signal that it's time to urinate). This final product contains all the waste that needs to be eliminated, while the correct amount of fluid and electrolytes remain, swirling perfectly balanced through the bloodstream.

Still awake? Good. Because along this meandering path, some intri-

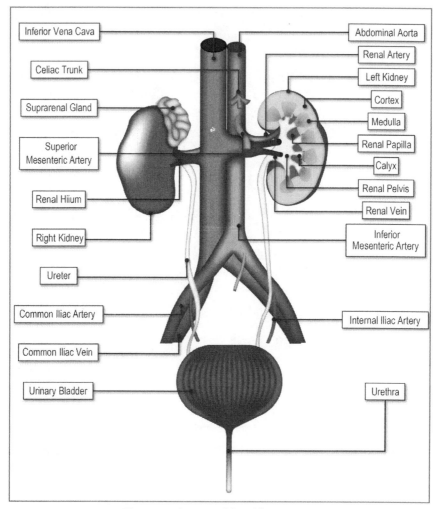

Figure 2: Diagram of the Kidney System

cate physiology occurs. Don't worry, I won't explain it all, other than to note that the dazzling brilliance of our body's physiology is nowhere better displayed than in each part of this tubular system.

For example, consider these two practical situations that require kidneys to either rid the body of excess water to prevent fluid overload or retain water to maintain blood pressure during severe dehydration.

First, imagine a person drinks a copious amount of water, say two quarts over a short period. Normal kidneys quickly respond by producing a large quantity of dilute urine resembling the ingested water, which exits the body through the urinary tract.

In fairness, the kidneys need a little help from their physiologic partner, the brain, to achieve this end. A region in the brain called the **hypothalamus** senses excess fluid in the blood and responds by turning off production of an anti-diuretic hormone (ADH), a hormone that prevents kidneys from excreting fluid. This allows the kidneys to produce large quantities of urine to rid the body of the excess water, preventing dangerous dilution of electrolytes in the blood, plus possible heart failure.

If that same person was stuck in Death Valley without water, dehydration would result. In this case, the hypothalamus would sense the fluid deficit and respond by secreting ADH to prevent further volume depletion and its life-threatening consequences. The kidneys, in turn, would respond to ADH by vigorously reabsorbing water, resulting in a reduced volume of (very concentrated) urine.

All this action unfolds in the nephron, that tiny unit of physiologic magic.

Kidneys are also endocrine organs, glands that secrete hormones essential for regulating bodily functions and maintaining good health. The idea of the kidney acting as an endocrine organ is relatively new, fully realized only during the past 35 years. This discovery and associated treatments developed to treat kidney disease and related abnormalities have profoundly assisted the preservation of ESRD patients' health. Here's an important clinical example: Kidney-disease patients inevitably experience enlarged parathyroid glands, of which there are four, located in the neck, under the thyroid gland (hence "para-thyroid"). They synthesize a hormone called parathormone (PTH). Renal failure causes an increase in PTH levels. Nephrologists are aware of and prepare for the myriad deleterious effects of excessive PTH. Nonetheless, controlling this symptom of kidney disease remains among the most difficult for patients and nephrologists alike.

One of my mentors, Dr. Shaul Massry, has written extensively about harm done to kidney-disease patients when PTH levels become too elevated. Co-edited by Dr. Richard Glassock of the renown, "Textbook of Nephrology," Dr. Massry calls PTH a "uremic toxin" that has a noxious effect on almost all organ systems. One of the more common and serious effects of secondary **hyperparathyroidism** (too much PTH) is severe bone disease. It may manifest with bone pain, muscle weakness, erosions in the bone cortex (outer portion) and osteoporosis. Elevated PTH can also cause severe itching, adding to dialysis patients' misery, and can accelerate cardiovascular disease (their most common cause of death) by enabling calcium to attach to artery walls, leading to heart attacks and gangrene.

Chronic renal failure also results in **hyperphosphatemia**, or dangerously high levels of phosphorus in the blood (a cruel cause-and- effect relationship links high phosphorus levels with high PTH levels). Unless a patient can significantly reduce intake of high-phosphate foods or bind the phosphorous in food with drugs that remove it from the intestine by bowel movement, phosphorus levels will continue to rise, contributing to morbidity and mortality.

Another important endocrine role of the kidney is synthesis of the active form of Vitamin D, necessary for bone health and for PTH to effectively normalize calcium and phosphorous levels in the blood. As the size of a diseased kidney shrinks, the amount of active Vitamin D it makes decreases, leaving a patient unable to properly absorb calcium in the intestinal tract. Low calcium levels, in turn, allow PTH to erode and weaken bones and enhance production of more PTH, a vicious cycle to say the least.

Still another vital kidney function is synthesis of **erythropoietin** (EPO), a protein responsible for maintenance of a normal red-blood-cell count (RBC). Red blood cells carry oxygen to all vital organs, and a low RBC causes anemia, that awful, foot-dragging, sluggish listlessness that makes you want to sleep for days. If coronary artery disease is present, anemia may also produce chest pain or angina.

Normal kidneys sense anemia and/or hypoxia (subnormal oxygen level), secreting EPO into the blood stream, which, when it reaches the bone marrow, corrects the deficiency by making new red blood cells. In chronic renal failure, the kidney cannot synthesize EPO and anemia just gets worse.

Kidneys are vital to maintaining normal blood pressure. Remember the one million nephrons per kidney, the ones that rid the body of excess salt and water? Well, when they're disease-damaged, salt and water are retained, increasing blood volume and with it, blood pressure. Initial treatment for a patient with newly diagnosed hypertension (above-normal blood pressure) includes reducing salt intake to decrease blood pressure. Drugs called diuretics ("water pills") can help rid the body of excess salt to control blood pressure as well.

Ultimately, dialysis helps regulate blood pressure by removing excess fluids (sometimes several liters per treatment), though patient compliance with a low-fluid, low-salt diet remains the best recipe for avoiding the dire consequences of hypertension—stroke, cardiac arrest, and death.

In some cases, as renal disease progresses, kidneys produce an excess of **angiotensin 2**, a powerful vasoconstrictor that also raises blood pressure to dangerous levels. Drugs called angiotensin-converting enzyme inhibitors (ACE) or angiotensin-receptor blockers (ARB) very effectively control this condition.

Then, there are the kidneys' effect on the gut.

Dr. Nick Vaziri, retired Professor Emeritus of Medicine, Physiology, and Biophysics at the University of California, Irvine, with whom I worked 40 years ago as renal fellows, shared with me several of his scientific papers covering diverse disciplines related to kidney diseases, ones he thought might be relevant to this book.

For example, another function of normal kidneys is to maintain a synergistic balance of the myriad bacteria species residing in the gastrointestinal tract. When the balance of trillions of bacteria is optimal, our immune system strengthens, our mood remains steady, and inflammation drops. As kidney disease progresses toward end-stage, however, the bacterial balance in our gut goes awry.

For example, when patients are fighting infections, they receive powerful broad-spectrum antibiotics that destroy not only "bad" bacteria causing the infection, but "good" protective species of gut flora, inducing the imbalance noted above.

In addition, we routinely tell patients to eat less fiber in the form of fruits and vegetables because they contain a lot of potassium. Sick kidneys are less able to remove potassium from the body and high levels may accumulate, inducing life-threatening situations. In a cruel, physiological irony (not the only one you'll read about in this book), the good bacteria depend on dietary fiber to thrive. Bacteria present in the GI tract, for example, are responsible for making serotonin, so necessary for good brain health. Too little may cause mood disorders like depression. Modern antidepressant drugs increase serotonin levels to optimize mood. Depression, so common in dialysis patients for obvious reasons— loss of organ function, job, sense of security, wellbeing, freedom to enjoy life, and eat and drink your favorites- now compounds because the brain doesn't receive adequate serotonin to help stabilize mood.

In a uremic environment, cells that line the colon develop a leak in a part of the cell called a "tight junction" (a minute passage between the cell and the internal milieu). This allows harmful bacterial products called endotoxins to pass into the system. Inflammatory substances also pass through these leaky junctions. Since inflammation plays a large role in producing cardiovascular disease in kidney patients (for whom it's the most common cause of death), repairing the cell, thereby preventing the leak, may remove an important element of the inflammatory state of chronic renal failure.

Dr. Vaziri calls this condition the "Intestinal Renal Syndrome" and works with nephrologists to test his hypothesis in ongoing clinical studies. Meanwhile, it seems that changing to a more plant-based, high-fiber diet may slow the progression to kidney failure, helping maintain crucial bacterial synergy and reducing the inflammatory nature of uremia.

In summary, unlike, say, lungs, whose main purpose is to provide oxygen and remove carbon dioxide, kidneys are highly complex organs that simultaneously multitask and perpetually regulate many bodily functions:

1. Nephrons maintain salt and water balance through filtration and tubular function;

2. Acid/base balance maintenance supports life;

3. Blood pressure control;

4. EPO regulates red-blood-cell count in response to anemia;

5. Kidneys activate Vitamin D;

6. Kidneys maintain normal phosphorus balance; and

7. Kidneys maintain normal gastrointestinal bacterial flora.

Treating ESRD

Chronic kidney failure progresses over considerable time, from inception to ESRD, and almost always involves both kidneys. Kidney disease itself is a silent, insidious predator. Over years, sometimes decades, it slowly destroys the organ's architecture, though patients typically don't feel ill until after losing about 70% of kidney function (a remarkably forgiving organ, but only to a point).

In fact, a patient might only realize they're sick—and how sick they really are—when a routine blood test reveals a **glomerular filtration rate** (GFR—the rate at which waste is filtered from the kidneys) of 30 cubic centimeters per minute or less. Normal GFR is well above 60cc/minute. At 30 cubic centimeters per minute, other indicators may confirm if kidney disease—any type of kidney disease that will ultimately shrink, scar and reduce the organ's function—is present.

Kidney disease is confirmed when lab tests show elevated levels of metabolic waste products, especially serum **creatinine** and **blood urea nitrogen (BUN)**, often accompanied by protein in the urine or clinically elevated blood pressure. Nephrologists can monitor a patient's kidney function and the rate at which function declines by following levels of these measurable substances.

As these levels rise, GFR falls, and when it dips below 15cc/min, **"uremic syndrome,"** a condition when kidneys cannot eliminate waste products, ensues.

Patients in this book all experienced uremic syndrome prior to beginning dialysis therapy. Symptoms included fatigue, insomnia, nausea, poor appetite, weight loss, inability to concentrate, confusion, depression, shortness of breath, bad breath, twitchiness, seizures, cramping, even coma.

One patient recalls, "I remember when I was severely uremic. My creatinine was 13 (normal is 0.6-1.4 milligrams per deciliter), my BUN was 160 (normal is 6 to 20 mg per 100 milliliters). I was swollen like a balloon, weak, wobbly, cramped like a bobby pin, walking into walls. My tongue was pale yellow (from retained nitrogen) and my thirst was unquenchable, on a par with chronic, unmitigated pain when it comes to physical discomfort. I didn't realize it then, but I was almost dead. Three doctors told me that in their cumulative careers, spanning 90 years, they'd never seen a uremic patient with those kinds of numbers still standing. Later, as I stabilized on dialysis, they let me in on a secret—they had nicknamed me 'the horse.'"

Patients aware of their chronic renal disease and followed by a nephrologist early in their illness, should never suffer this kind of life-threatening uremia. Early detection with timely referral to a nephrologist makes a huge difference. Education, prevention of secondary hyperparathyroidism, using EPO to avert severe anemia, medicating for blood pressure control, even early intervention with dialysis—all these weapons populate the nephrologist's arsenal.

Because some intact, individual nephrons can overachieve, adapting to renal injury by a process of "hyper-filtration," early stages of kidney disease are often quite subtle. Stage 2 exhibits a mildly reduced GFR of 60-89cc/min. Stage three hits when GFR drops to 30-59cc/min. Stage 4 is when most kidney disease can be identified by rising blood creatinine and BUN, but a patient still feels well. Stage 5 is defined by a GFR less than 15cc/min and is usually associated with elements of uremic syndrome. Medical intervention and dialysis are treatments of choice, unless a preemptive renal transplant occurs, which, by orders of magnitude, is the best therapy of all.

"I remember being told a kidney transplant was one of several therapeutic options," recalls a patient who spent considerable time on dialysis. "That may be the lingo, but once I got the kidney, I realized it was not a therapeutic option, at least not like other options. It was a new life."

I pause to preach: We can prevent or attenuate so many illnesses by simply having an annual physical exam, discussing results with our doctor, along with family history and any new bit of information that seems strange or abnormal about our health.

Consider early cancer detection. I'm a perfect example of how early detection of lung cancer, revealed by a chest x-ray, gave me a chance to survive. Baseline blood tests are equally critical for early detection of kidney disease. Elevated blood pressure, for example, should lead to a thorough investigation of cause. Though certainly not always, it could signify early kidney disease, or, if treated, help prevent it. A urinalysis showing protein in the urine of an otherwise healthy person might indicate early kidney disease. Blood tests may confirm a patient has stage 3 chronic renal disease. Knowledge is king and can save your life, so consider this a universal prescription: Annual routine blood and urine tests and a visit to the doctor.

Detecting kidney disease early also helps mitigate many consequences of the disease, like **secondary hyperparathyroidism** and **Vitamin D** deficiency, which can be addressed by reducing the amount of dietary phosphorus consumed, especially from foods like dairy, eggs and protein in general. Adding the active form of Vitamin D, available in a pill, helps reduce stimulus of the parathyroid glands to make PTH. A phosphorus binder, discussed earlier, can help when diet alone isn't enough to normalize the level. For more advanced secondary hyperparathyroidism, Sensipar, a drug that lowers PTH levels and protects a patient's bones, is often prescribed.

Despite our best efforts, most patients with chronic kidney disease already exhibit significant hyperparathyroidism by the time nephrologists see them. When an ESRD patient requires dialysis, reducing phosphorus levels can be a hellish challenge. As if being so sick wasn't enough, now they need to excel as amateur nutritionists, spending hours learning what they can and cannot eat, including cutting out high-phosphorus foods like cheese, milk, and ice cream—sources of near-universal culinary pleasure.

And since all high-protein foods contain phosphorus, normalizing phosphorous levels is virtually impossible by diet alone. Adding to patients' confusion, they're also told protein intake is necessary for good nutrition.

Despite repeated dietary instructions, patients say they rarely remembered the message or fully understood its significance until several months into dialysis. Even then, when the message resonated, it meant losing more of the little things that make life enjoyable.

For new dialysis patients, having just left the hospital confused and frightened about their condition and their future, life is one giant oxymoron. You need nutrition, but don't eat all this nutritious stuff. You're thirsty as hell, but with diminished urination, don't drink because you'll retain that fluid, sending your blood pressure off the chart. And remember to dutifully take a dizzying array of medications at the right time in the right dosage. Just swallowing the meds might require all the fluid you're allowed for one day.

These physical and emotional challenges, along with feeling crappy much of the time and spending nine hours a week tethered like a prisoner to a life-sustaining dialysis machine, can drag patient, family, friends, and loved ones into a quagmire of gloom.

Could it be more arduous, could more simple pleasures disappear? Unfortunately, yes. Levels of potassium, an electrolyte essential to life and regulated by healthy kidneys, can, if unmanaged, rise dramatically with ESRD. High potassium levels can cause severe muscle weakness and extra heartbeats. If they rise even higher, life-threatening cardiac abnormalities can occur, including cessation of heart beat or cardiac arrest and death—stark but important news for any dialysis patient, terrifying for those with existing heart disease.

Potassium-rich foods include more of the consumables we love, foods we normally consider "healthy," like fruits, especially citrus, berries, avocados, grapes and bananas.

Now for the good news: If a patient meets headlong the challenges of healthy living with ESRD, it gets a little easier because they feel physically and emotionally better with tighter fluid balance and proper maintenance of phosphorus and potassium levels. Some continue working full-time, and many can enjoy light physical activity central to their "former" lives.

Hemodialysis

So, what is dialysis, the ultimate maintenance tool for ESRD patients, like? For now, we'll focus on the most common type of dialysis, hemodialysis.

Most often, initial treatments require placement of a catheter into a large vein from which the patient's blood can flow through an artificial kidney to be cleansed of toxic wastes. Although considered a minor procedure by radiologists who do it often and do it well, for the terrified, uremic patient, it's a big deal, an invasive procedure that carries risk. Later during the treatment course, the same patient will require another surgery to create an **arteriovenous fistula** (A-V fistula, a connection between an artery and a vein, typically in the forearm). that provides a permanent access site for ongoing hemodialysis treatments. I had one patient who kept his catheter, which twice needed replacement, for two years. For him, the A-V fistula was a sign of giving in, a sign of permanent resignation to life on dialysis. Eventually, he got the kidney transplant he envisioned and fought for.

ESRD and dialysis also mean loss, like loss of work and income, inextricably linked to identity, self-esteem, and security. For some, it's loss of sexual interest or relations. For families, it tears at the tapestry of our closest relations. It can destroy marriages. Strong unions, in which

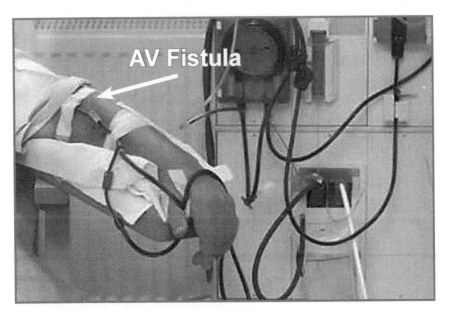

AV fistula

a partner can participate in patient care while maintaining their own purpose, identity, and sense of "self," stand the best chance of enduring.

Not surprising, then, that many dialysis patients take anti-depression medications. Also not surprising, patients strong enough to cope with dialysis, comply with its regimen and maintain optimism and hope for the future are the ones who, barring physiological barriers, make the best transplant candidates, ultimately pushing through to a new lease on life.

But getting there isn't easy and often not quick. There are no ruby slippers. Many dialysis patients must buckle in for a long, arduous ride. Dietary and fluid restrictions are daunting enough for a day, let alone months or years. Sitting thrice weekly in a chair, watching your blood swirl through an artificial kidney for hours at a time, is depressing, even surrealistic, an image from a Dali painting.

Patients develop strong bonds with each other, maybe the strongest bonds they enjoy, lying there, bound by circumstance, needles, and tubes. And loss is always in the air. A patient's death, for example, devastates all. When "Joe" misses a couple of treatments, other patients know there are only two likely reasons—he's in the hospital for specialized care or he's gone. Gone for good.

Some patients, especially older ones, ask themselves, "What purpose am I serving? Is there sufficient meaning in my life to justify the suffering?"

Discussions I've had with patients who wished to talk about purpose, meaning, and spirituality, to decide whether they wanted to continue dialysis, have taught me to be patient, a good listener and hopeful. Over time, some patients began to feel physically better with treatment. Accompanied by diminishing anxiety and depression, their dark view of life lightens, and they rediscover purpose. It could be family, intellectual growth, companionship, or the simple delight of tending a home garden. There are as many reasons as there are patients who rebound from depression and carry on.

Dr. Lionel Corbett, recognized expert in Jungian therapy and author of *The Soul in Anguish*, concludes, "At times, the discovery of meaning in suffering is closely tied to the meaning we have always attributed to our life, but at other times radically new meaning may emerge. Suffering or a life crisis can therefore provide important developmental possibilities."

Our renal health-care team understands this principal and gives sufficient support to help patients navigate emotional roadblocks. As a result, many of our patients receive transplants or life-meaning on dialysis.

Nephrologists, nurses, dieticians, and social workers function as a team, wearing coach and cheerleader caps to encourage patient compliance with the litany of lifestyle restrictions, conveying the message that a renal transplant or, if that is not possible, an active, satisfying life, is possible. It's undertaken with respect and understanding of each patient's character strengths and weaknesses, which also takes time.

But it's tricky work that goes beyond just managing dialysis treatments and the considerable work of understanding renal physiology. Consider what this patient told me: "The one thing that pisses me off most is baby-talk, as if because I'm on dialysis and can't walk around like normal folks, I'm a dependent child, unable to understand basic concepts of nutrition and health care. Speak to me like an adult, for God's sake."

Fortunately, that incident did not occur in our unit, but sadly and predictably, the message resonates. Dialysis patients are people who bleed red and cry salty tears like everybody else. Treat them respectfully, like family, and treat *their families*, so indispensable to this complicated partnership, the same. Educate, encourage, and listen—hallmarks of good patient care and defining characteristics of our staff at the Santa Barbara Artificial Kidney Center, where medicine is equal parts science and art. I call it the marriage of "High Tech" and "High Touch."

But still there remain myriad challenges with dialysis treatments themselves. Sure, there's the difficult work of precisely setting a dialysis machine to remove the correct amount of potassium and fluid to achieve exceptional lab results. But even "good numbers" can deceive, not always reflecting how a patient "feels." For example, like soldiers who develop Post Traumatic Stress Disorder (PTSD) returning, from, say, Iraq, dialysis patients may have normal blood chemistries, but are emotionally wounded, perhaps for life, by inescapable anguish. Wellness, then, cannot always be measured from a blood test alone and must be addressed by the entire health-care team for a patient to thrive. Psychiatric referrals, for patients and their families are often part of this mix.

Nurses often double as mental-health support as well. Rather than just informing a patient about weight, blood pressure, phosphorous, and potassium levels, they ask questions that provide an emotional forum to share internalized anxieties and frustrations. My patients tell me they appreciate that our staff finds time during a very challenging day to see them as human beings who feel lost, confused, frightened, and need explanations. Doing so, they inspire hope for a healthier future.

Here's a example of what happens when the whole team—head nurse, physician assistant, social worker, nutritionist and nephrologist—meet to discuss each patient's progress and draft plans on moving forward. We were recently discussing a patient who had been on dialysis for about four years and was on the transplant list, but was beginning to "fail to thrive." His serum potassium levels were slowly rising, demonstrating an attitude of, *"So what if I die from a cardiac arrest?"* Psychiatrists consider this a suicidal gesture. The patient was frustrated, lonely, and had lost everything that was meaningful in his life (you'll read his stranger-than-fiction story later). Our job was to prevent him from committing suicide by non-compliance (high potassium), provide hope, and get him to the "transplant promised land."

Peritoneal Dialysis

So far, I've discussed only one form of renal replacement therapy, hemodialysis. Another form of dialysis, peritoneal dialysis (PD), is performed at home and offers many advantages for a patient who masters the procedure. Usually the patient who chooses PD is independent-minded, generally healthier, more proactive, younger, and might work full time.

What is peritoneal dialysis? It's based on elementary principles of chemistry, namely osmosis and diffusion, and utilizes the semi-permeable membrane, called the peritoneum, that lines the abdominal cavity, Some substances can pass through the membrane, others cannot. Blood from an ESRD patient contains high concentrations of Blood Urea Ni-

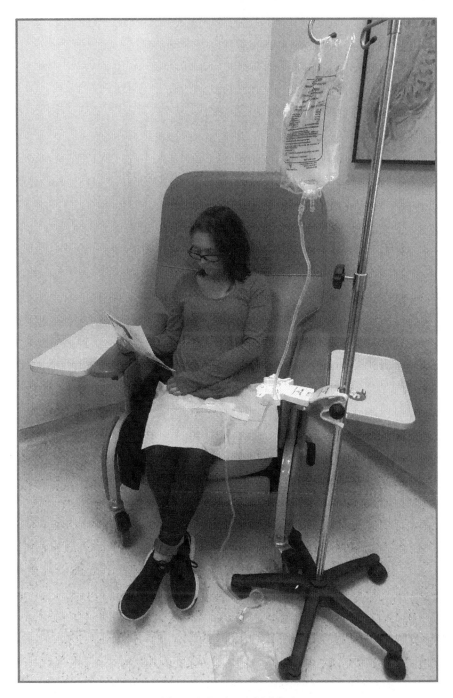

Figure 3: Peritoneal Dialysis

trogen (BUN, described earlier). It circulates through the many small blood vessels in the semi-permeable peritoneum. If fluid containing no BUN were allowed to bathe this membrane over time, the BUN would come out of the blood and into the fluid that contains no BUN. This tendency for molecules to move from an area of higher concentration to an area of lower concentration is called diffusion. If this same fluid contained a high concentration of glucose, it would pull water from blood vessels of the peritoneum into the fluid. This is the process of osmosis, the passage of less concentrated fluid across a semi-permeable membrane into a more concentrated one.

Using this principle, a small catheter is surgically placed within the peritoneal membrane in the lower abdomen. The patient generally leaves the hospital the same day or the next morning. The catheter is literally in touch with the intestine. It is ready to go in 7-10 days.

The patient attends classes at the Santa Barbara Artificial Kidney Center, learning how to deliver a specially designed fluid called **dialysate**, containing various concentrations of glucose (sugar), into the tube that was surgically placed in the peritoneal membrane. The higher the glucose concentration, the larger the quantity of water it will draw out of the blood and into the cavity. Fluid dwells in the cavity, always in contact with small blood vessels in the peritoneal membrane, for a period of time. This allows toxins like BUN, creatinine and others, plus excess accumulated water, to cross the membrane and remain in the peritoneal cavity. Utilizing gravity, the bag is lowered so that the fluid drains out of the abdomen and into the bag and is eventually discarded.

Some patients can perform this procedure before going to sleep by utilizing a computerized device that allows the appropriate amount of fluid to enter the peritoneal cavity, dwell, then drain into a bag to be discarded when the patient awakens. The patient disconnects the tube coming out of his or her abdomen using sterile technique, then tapes the small flexible tube to the abdomen and goes about their day. This type of dialysis is called **continuous cyclic peritoneal dialysis** (CCPD). Alternatively, some patients would rather do the exchanges manually four or five times a day. This is called chronic ambulatory peritoneal dialysis (CAPD).

Dr. Carl Kjellstrand, who received the annual Lifetime Achievement in Hemodialysis award in 2014, coined the term the "unphysiology of dialysis." He asserted that many side effects of hemodialysis were related to inadequate duration and frequency of the procedure. Peritoneal dialysis, on the other hand, while not quite up to the work of our native kidneys, is more "physiologic" because it can be performed with greater frequency and duration.

Patients who choose P.D. are more likely to take ownership and control of their illness, shedding dependence on the nursing staff and the dialysis machine. In addition, peritoneal dailysis patients frequently can continue to work, exercise, eat, and drink with less restriction, and take back some control of their lives. Because the procedure is done seven days a week, patients have fewer fluid and food restrictions. These patients have less depression and anxiety and, unless they have frequent attacks of peritonitis (infection of the peritoneal membrane), have a less daunting road to renal transplantation.

Kidney Transplantation–The Holy Grail

The third form of replacement therapy, and by far the best, is renal transplantation.

Kidney transplants are far more successful today than they used to be, due to better understanding of the immune system, new anti-rejection medications, better surgical techniques, and the willingness of living donors to step forward. (Introducing healthy transplant recipients to dialysis patients inspires patients to persevere and overcome adversity. A way of "passing it forward," so to speak, offering hope to those who need it most.)

Dialysis, in fact, is not always necessary for an ESRD patient or soon-to-be ESRD patient. A nephrologist follows the patient closely, and along the way, while applying strategies to slow the advance of renal disease, educates the patient about available remedies, including transplantation.

When the patient's GFR approaches 30cc/min, it's time to explore a preemptive renal transplant, while the patient is symptom-free and in the best physical shape to receive one. Due to advances in genetic matching, unrelated donors like a spouse or friend may be good candidates to donate, not to mention candidates often closely matched to the patient—family members like mothers, fathers, sisters, and brothers.

These days, many dialysis patients turn to social-media platforms to "get the word out" about their plight. When friends and associates (work, church, gym members, social clubs) who may not know the patient needs a transplant, receive a text, tweet or Facebook post, they can respond directly or spread the word with a single keystroke, increasing the pool of persons "in the know." In the end, it's amazing who steps forward to donate. It seems, blessedly, there's usually "one in every crowd." The key is building that crowd, and patients are getting better at it.

The complex, time-consuming process of evaluating the patient and potential donors begins with a call to the transplant center, where immunologic testing of patient and potential donor, as well as psychological evaluation of both, are performed. We're blessed to have Cedars Sinai Medical Center in Los Angeles as our transplant partner.

If a living-donor transplant is not immediately feasible, the average waiting period for a "deceased" or "cadaveric" kidney is 4-8 years. Dialysis patients need to "hang in there" and comply with outrageously austere lifestyle demands to remain healthy enough to receive that transplant. It takes immeasurable focus, patience, and determination, but the payoff is huge, often resulting in return to a normal, healthy life. It's all about "stick and stay and make it pay"—a mantra for patients pursuing transplantation.

Unlike the slow, creeping drumbeat of declining kidney function, results of a transplant are often nearly immediate. Once a new kidney is placed in the recipient, "pinks up" with renewed blood flow and begins pumping out urine, creatinine and BUN levels plummet.

Consider this from one transplant patient. "I couldn't believe it, but my creatinine went from 7 to 1.4 four days after surgery. I specifically remember waking up before dawn on the third day. Sure, I was sore from surgery, but I could immediately feel that I was well again. I asked the nurse for a favor—to open the blinds of my hospital room so I could watch the sunrise. After all, a new day was dawning."

Arresting Kidney Disease

By now you know about the complex, intricate role kidneys play in maintaining our health and wellbeing, and the chaos caused when they fail. That said, the extreme state of uremic syndrome described earlier, should, in the 21st century, never occur. Even though all the nephrologist's tools can't completely arrest the relentless progression of nephron loss, in many cases they can slow its decline and prevent a cascade of other complications such as cardiac disease, especially when kidney disease is diagnosed early.

So, what tools do they employ to accomplish this?

1. **Controlling blood pressure** with angiotensin converting enzyme (ACE) inhibitors, angiotensin receptor blockers (ARB), and/or diuretics ("water pills").

2. **Treating high cholesterol** with appropriate diet and a statin drug helps prevent coronary artery disease, which so often accompanies kidney failure, especially in diabetic patients. In addition, it may slow deterioration of kidney function.

3. **Maintaining perfect blood sugar for a patient with diabetes**, the most common cause of kidney failure worldwide. Uncontrolled diabetes can lead to well-known complications— blindness, neuropathy, heart disease, amputations, and, of course, kidney failure.

4. **Modestly reducing protein intake**, especially from high-phosphorous dairy products. That said, a delicate balance of protein intake must be achieved, especially in patients who lose lots of protein in their urine. (**Nephrotic Syndrome**, a condition that may herald many different kidney diseases, is associated with large urinary protein loss. You will read about a patient who presented with the nephrotic syndrome and was ultimately diagnosed correctly, but not until after considerable torment).

5. **Educating the patient** about drugs and supplements that may harm the kidneys, especially when a multibillion dollar industry attracts frightened people who may be in denial about

their illness or who had a bad medical experience—either of which can undermine critical thinking. Blinded by myth and seduced by promises of miracle cures, which might be harmless snake-oil products, or, worse, may damage already-compromised kidneys, some will try almost anything to get well.

Impure Chinese herbs, for example, can cause kidney failure. Or consider this: non-steroid, anti-inflammatory drugs (NSAIDS) can be bought over the counter. In general, they're useful for relieving minor arthritic pain or headache. Used in larger amounts in kidney-disease patients, they can accelerate renal failure. Physicians must find time to listen to their patients and credibly explain the do's and don'ts of diet and self-medication.

6. **Maintaining adequate hydration,** as counterintuitive as it seems, is important for renal patients, especially in the early phases of kidney disease. Some lose salt and water because of their disease and require more intake. Fluid loss from any cause can worsen kidney function. In conjunction with NSAIDS the combination is particularly "nephrotoxic."

7. **Special attention is always warranted with older patients,** because aging itself is a form of chronic renal disease. As we age, nephrons become "obsolescent," a fancy word pathologists use to define old nephrons seen on a kidney biopsy. The elderly are more prone to acute renal injury than a younger folks. Dosages of drugs metabolized by the kidney must be appropriately adjusted for age.

Now, let's look at some patients who leaned in and battled kidney disease with every morsel of strength they could muster.

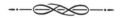

Chapter 3

Sarah

Not long ago, Sarah, a friend and a patient, called me from the Los Angeles Airport because she forgot a doctor's note explaining why her dog, Big Ed, should be allowed to accompany her on a flight to Paris. I quickly wrote an email explaining that Sarah was a renal transplant patient, who depended on Big Ed to allay chronic anxiety. Fortunately, the officials of the airline accepted it. Sarah boarded the plane with Big Ed buckled in with her, and they crossed the Atlantic together.

For the others in the plane, it may have just been one more trans-oceanic flight, but to Sarah, it was the trip of a lifetime. To understand just how improbable this Paris trip was for her, we need to climb into a time machine and go back to her childhood, when the upheaval of her parent's bitter divorce may have initiated a chain-reaction of life-threatening events.

When Sarah was six years old, her parents split up after a 13-year marriage. "They were impossibly young, and had four children, all girls, one after the other," Sarah explains. "It was very hard on my mother, who postponed her career to raise the kids. Dad, meanwhile, was pursuing a career in academics. He'd received a PhD in mathematics and was working toward a second in philosophy.

Sarah's dad, Bill, was a tenured professor at the University of Indiana who accepted a one year visiting professorship in the department of mathematics at UCSB. In August, 1975, Susan, Bill and their four daughters, packed up what they needed for a year and moved to Santa Barbara. Bill told me that they were having marital problems while living in Indiana and that he hoped that the change of venue would provide a new a chance to work out their difficulties in Santa Barbara. The promise of beautiful beaches and working at a university with views of the Pacific was alluring. However, he had no illusions about the challenges to come and they had both agreed to seek the help of marriage counseling at the Family and Children's Center in Santa Barbara. They spent that academic year in weekly counselling sessions with the center's therapist. As the year came to a close, Bill felt slightly optimistic that the marriage could be saved.

In May 1976 Bill went back to Indiana to teach summer school with the understanding that he would return to Santa Barbara at the end of the summer and then the family would all move back to Indiana together. "On my return to Santa Barbara, Susan informed me that she did not think that the marriage could work and that she would prefer to stay in Santa Barbara with the four children." Bill felt that even if the marriage was lost, that they needed to at least return to Indiana as a family and work out the logistics of the situation. Bill's income was completely generated from his tenured appointment at the University of Indiana and were the only funds available to support the family. Bill pondered why would Susan not want to go back and settle all of the complex legal and financial arrangements. Bill was stunned when he was abruptly served with divorce papers. To add to this depressing story, the therapist from the Family and Children's Center soon moved in with Susan and the children.

Sarah, the second daughter, felt a tremendous loss when her dad, moved back to Bloomington, Indiana to resume his job teaching math at Indiana University. The children thought they were going back together. There was tremendous confusion, anxiety and fear within each child. It was not possible for them to comprehend a stranger living in their home, replacing their dad, with no acceptable explanation. The seeds of disease had been placed within the children in the form of unbearable stress and trauma!

She recognizes now that divorce for them was a better alternative to staying together. But, she never fully recovered from the traumatic separation that shredded her family, leaving her mom to raise her sisters alone.

Sarah was never completely healthy after that. She suffered a variety of minor infections and frequent colds and finally, a couple of years later, she began experiencing an uncomfortable and persistent fever. Her doctor assured her it was a just viral infection that would likely get better with time. It turned out to be a misdiagnosis. Sarah continued to feel worse and then began suffering from joint pain and that was followed by an odd, frightening facial rash. She underwent a series of blood tests, which revealed she was suffering from something more serious than a viral infection. One of the tests, called an anti-nuclear antibody, or ANA, was strongly positive. It meant her immune system was malfunctioning and attacking her own tissue. Other sophisticated tests confirmed a diagnosis of Systemic Lupus Erythematosus (SLE, or Lupus, for short). Sarah and her mother were devastated. Bill was equally affected, saddened and frustrated that Sarah had such a cryptic diagnosis. They were told her future would be filled with long and chronic health battles, with wide-ranging symptoms. They were shocked and dismayed, but even that sober diagnosis did not fully paint the picture of what was to come.

Sarah's mother, Susan, had a will of iron, though, and an indomitable maternal spirit. Even when Sarah was diagnosed with this extremely complex and dangerous disease, Susan accepted the challenge like a tigress defending her young.

A rheumatologist told Susan that her Sarah needed to start on corticosteroids immediately. These powerful, anti-inflammatory drugs can be very effective, but they also can cause many serious side-effects. Used for a short period to treat, say, an allergic reaction, then tapered and discontinued, they're generally safe and effective. The same, however, isn't true when you depend on them over months and years to quiet painful, inflamed joints. With continued use over time, a patient develops a rounded face ("Cushingoid Syndrome"), extra fatty tissue over the upper neck, weight gain, excessive appetite, and acne. The brain changes, too, sometimes causing depression, insomnia, even psychosis. Over time, the patient may develop diabetes, hypertension, bone disease, adrenal insufficiency, and a predisposition to infections. It can cause tremendous mood swings, from depression to anxiety to great burst of anger.

Sarah was only a teenager when all this came bearing down on her. Adolescence itself, of course, is uniquely challenging and turbulent. Even for a healthy teen, it's a time of disorientation and discovery, a time when peer groups exert pressure and often behave cruelly. An interest in sex develops and external appearances become critical to social success. And since the brain's frontal lobes, which are associated with, among other things, reward and attention, don't fully develop until our mid-twenties, teenagers, in the words of rock legend Bob Seger, often find themselves, "Workin' on mysteries without any clues."

Sarah's world was full of confusion and pressure. Besides suffering through her parents' divorce and her debilitating illness, money was tight. Her mother, while trying to stay at home with the children as much as possible, still had to work part-time to provide essentials for her family. She was sometimes at work when Sarah needed her the most. The emotional toll on Sarah mounted.

She was taking a number of steroids to reduce symptoms and induce remission. During those years of treatment with high-dose steroids, she had countless blood draws and doctor appointments. She suffered waxing and waning disease symptoms. She finally began to respond clinically to medication, with less joint pain, rash, and fatigue, but she was exhausted and struggled emotionally.

With this relief came a terrible tradeoff—the troubling side effects of cortisone. Sarah gained weight and was beset by redistributed fatty tissue around her neck. She developed acne and her face got round. Her mood became labile and surly. She felt ugly, ashamed of her appearance, and confused. In retrospect, she says, "I felt like a freak of nature running on the treadmill of life, desperately trying to find the person I'd once been."

Her mother agonized over her daughter's extreme discomfort. Susan bathed Sarah with unconditional love and support, but filled with cortisone, Sarah had episodes of anger and cursed the medicine that changed her body from a thin, pretty teenager into the 'hideous creature' she saw in the mirror. These outbursts emotionally drained Susan, who was constantly challenged with how she should react. There are few guidebooks to raising a child with these kinds of health issues, not to mention the incredible array of side-effects from the medicines. Susan felt like she was alone in every decision she made about her daughter. She chose to allow Sarah to scream and externalize her feelings, but continued to talk quietly with her, whenever Sarah was receptive, about all the reasons Sarah needed to take her meds. She always offered her daughter hope for better times to come. When words failed, Susan simply held her and hugged her tight.

As often occurs in families that suffer from kidney and other serious health issues, the dynamics can get confusing. For example, Sarah's younger sister, Nina, remembers resenting Sarah, who always took center stage at home. Despite Sarah's horrible travails, Nina felt her sister was dominating her mother's attention and she felt unnoticed and insignificant. Her feelings are often mirrored by the young siblings of chronic disease sufferers. It is part of the often complex emotional tremors that can shake families to the core. Love, understanding, constant positive communication and a strong spiritual belief are all part of making it through this – as well as the feeling that no matter how difficult it is, the family will come out of it intact. It tests everyone, from the children to the parents. Sarah's family was a wonderful example of how this challenge can be met. Nina, for example, despite her anger and ambivalence back then, began to understand the situation as she grew older and today she is a loving sister, who still stands by Sarah in times of need.

For the next few years, Sarah took high doses of prednisone, an oral corticosteroid, when her disease would flare up. After symptoms improved, dosage was tapered, but Sarah was never off steroids altogether. Other drugs were also added to fix her out-of-control immune system. Her illness was stubborn and always required a cocktail of powerful drugs to manage it.

A beautiful, intelligent, and talented girl, Sarah was blessed with the gift of an exceptional voice. She dreamed of becoming an actor or professional singer, but her illness sapped her hope and made her feel like that dream was unobtainable, just a fantasy. She entered high school and her experience there was miserable. Socially, she felt like a misfit, unable to concentrate on her studies. Her life revolved around her illness, with its fluctuating symptoms, medical monitoring and periods of self-loathing. While others went to the prom or out to parties, she often went to the hospital for treatment.

Predictably, with the combination of teenage hormones and the sometimes terrible effects of steroids, Sarah's behavior grew increasingly bizarre. By age 16, her mood swings were intense, and at times she'd erupt in profane rants toward her mother and everyone else around her. F-bombs rained down like mortars. She even blamed her mother for her illness. Of course, this type of erratic behavior and rage is often consistent with excess steroid use. Susan knew it was the Lupus and its treatments talking, but nonetheless she felt the full weight of a mother's lament and a haunting guilt that she couldn't do better for her daughter. In a ripple effect, all family members suffered. Susan felt as if she was treading water, trying to stay afloat, absorbing each new challenge, determined to protect her kids. With only so much time in a day, she often had none left for listening to and comforting Sarah's sisters, who resented Sarah for the non-stop attention she got.

One night, Sarah was having dinner with family and friends at a restaurant when she suddenly stood up and started singing. It was bizarre behavior and Susan did her best to cover for her daughter by acting as it if was a big joke, but she knew her daughter was in trouble. Shortly after, at a dinner with friends, Sarah made a huge scene, scaring everyone present and Susan rushed her to the emergency room. Diagnosed with psychosis, Sarah was admitted to Cottage Hospital's Psychiatric Unit, where she remained for several months until her illness, caused by acute brain inflammation, was controlled.

Sarah was given intravenous infusions of very high-dose corticosteroids, (which, ironically, caused the problem in the first place), and to balance this, she was given anti-psychotic medication and anti-depressants. She continued to take oral steroids and a drug called Imuran to control her Lupus. Only 16 years old at the time of her psychotic break, Sarah was at the peak of adolescent hormonal changes, characterized by high levels of estrogen, which themselves can cause Lupus flare-ups. It bears repeating that corticosteroids can also wreak havoc with the brain and cause the very symptoms that resulted in Sarah's admission to a locked psychiatric unit.

Finally, Sarah was well enough to return home, though Susan and her other daughters were enervated and bone-weary. It was then decided that Sarah would benefit by spending time with her dad in Indiana. He took excellent care of her over the next three years, and with his guidance, she passed her General Educational Development exams and enrolled in Indiana University's School of Drama.

During this time, Sarah's optimism returned. She felt hopeful for the first time since Lupus turned her life upside down. She believed she was back on course to follow her dream of becoming an actor. Her Lupus remained controlled and her mood improved without need of medication.

Toward the end of her third year living with her dad, however, Sarah noticed some ankle swelling. A urinalysis revealed protein, and she was referred to a nephrologist. She was told the unhappy news, her kidney function was abnormal, showing elevated levels of creatinine and BUN, those classic markers of decreased kidney function.

A renal biopsy revealed Lupus Nephritis, an inflammation of the kidneys brought on by her primary disease. Sarah took a diuretic for the swelling in her legs and was told to remain on her dose of prednisone and Imuran. At the time, she felt well and would not have known there was a problem if not for the ankle swelling.

She was devastated by the news. It seemed as though she was getting better and now this terrible turn. She was buoyed by her family and she began to try to just take one day at a time. She returned to her mother's home in Santa Barbara six months after the biopsy. She wasn't giving up. She decided to pursue opportunities in drama and reunite with her family. Looking back, she now admits that during this time, she was unaware of the true gravity of her situation. It was during this time that she was referred to me for ankle swelling and further clarification of her kidney issues. When I reviewed Sarah's records it was clear she'd had Lupus Nephritis for many years, manifested by minimal protein in prior urine samples. Although her Lupus was quite aggressive on her initial admission to Cottage Hospital as a teenager, her kidneys had not, at the time, indicated loss of filtering ability. But Lupus plays by its own, bizarre rules. In some cases, there can be complete remission, but in others, such as Sarah's, it can lie dormant, then awaken like a dragon and quickly damage organs. Her body's ability to filter waste products was suddenly and severely impaired. Her blood pressure elevated, consistent with kidney involvement, and this required more drugs to control it. She was losing large amounts of protein in her urine, consistent with nephrotic syndrome. In addition, she had the anemia of chronic kidney failure. Many other blood-test results were abnormal and consistent with chronic renal failure. An ultrasound revealed what I already knew, she had small, sick kidneys.

Sarah's life was about to take another dramatic turn, but not the kind of drama she so dearly loved. She knew that she was not well, but was unaware she had ESRD and would soon need dialysis. I had to explain this to her. We spent a long time together while I slowly outline the fact that there was no cure for this illness, but with dialysis she would soon feel better, and over time she would be an excellent candidate for a kidney transplant. Sarah initially denied her symptoms, but during our talk, she admitted she felt weak, cold and intermittently nauseous—all manifestations of chronic renal failure. When I suggested she start dialysis soon, she broke down and cried in my arms.

Sarah was only 20 years old when we met. She asked many questions about a possible transplant and tried to answer in an upbeat way. I was now her physician and coach – which is the way it should be, I might add. I indicated that the treatment to maintain a kidney transplant and to prevent rejection was the same as for Lupus. This included strict compliance with medications, including steroids. I pointed out that many Lupus patients, who received kidney transplants, not only succeeded with the new organ, but achieved complete remission of their primary disease.

To this day, Sarah remembers our conversation well because the hope she gathered from it was important impetus for her to embrace dialysis as a means to an end. Within a week, surgeons placed a vascular catheter in a subclavian vein and she began hemodialysis treatments. I had promised her she would feel better, and she did. Her weight came down as we removed liters of extra fluid. She could see the shape of her ankles again, and with erythropoietin injections, her anemia corrected and her energy level rose.

The 'honeymoon' period, was brief, however. Soon after starting dialysis, she described herself as "tethered to a machine like a prisoner, with no possible escape." Her family discussed possible candidates for donating a kidney. Because the sisters were so young, they were initially ruled out, so Susan offered to donate. Such a thing can never be fully appreciated, even if it is a mother donating a kidney to one of her children. It is heroic, beautiful and one of the most inspiring things I've ever experienced. The doctors cleared the operation and the rise in Sarah's spirits was amazing to watch. She had hope again. Her mother was positive during the entire process, never indicating she had any doubts about the procedure. Kidney donation was – and is – among the highest and most self-less actions a human being can take. I am always awed and filled with an immense sense of a love for humanity when a donation takes place.

The operation went smoothly. Everyone was exhausted, but exhilarated. Susan was tremendously excited for her daughter and felt she had done everything possible, which, of course, she had. Sarah immediately went through a period where her health was better than it had been in years. Her new kidney worked well and it eliminated many of the worst symptoms that she been suffering. It also kept her off dialysis. She was thrilled.

The transplant occurred in 1990, and in those days, a donor underwent surgery that necessitated a large incision in the flank, cutting through muscles to remove the kidney, resulting in significant post-operative pain. Susan still has a huge scar that reminds her of that ordeal. Like many donors back in the day, she sports it like a badge of honor, though. In my view, it is an amazingly special and is equivalent to the Medal of Honor given to our soldiers for valor. I can't think of anyone who deserves this kind of recognition more than living kidney donors.

From the very beginning of Sarah's post-transplant life, however, her kidney function was imperfect. There was, unfortunately, no effective induction therapy at the time. Today we have ways of helping patients ward off rejection and that vastly improve the longevity of renal transplants. Also, there were fewer immunosuppressant drugs, making it less likely a transplanted kidney would endure.

After a time, the gradual and progressive loss of Sarah's kidney function grew evident, and as her creatinine levels relentlessly climbed. The thought of again needing dialysis treatments made her sad and angry. "How could my own mother's kidney fail?" she asked herself again and again. Her mother was devastated, too. She felt like her kidney wasn't good enough.

Sarah landed back on dialysis, sitting for four hours at a time, three days a week, watching her blood circulate through the artificial kidney and return to her body, free of toxic waste products. Unfortunately, there is no similar treatment for lifting her spirits from her toxic, emotional morass.

Once we began earnestly discussing ways to move quickly toward a second kidney transplant, however, Sarah perked up. The medicinal value of hope, though not evident in blood tests, is astonishingly powerful. I could see it in Sarah's eyes. She appeared to me to be in a place where she could make an emotional move toward wellness.

Again, kidney-center staff remained upbeat, encouraging Sarah to follow their directions and get into great condition for transplant number two. She was put on the list for a deceased patient donor and waited. She was not on the list for long before a kidney that seemed an exceptional match, became available.

Sarah's family transported her quickly to Cedars Sinai, where she underwent her second kidney transplant. Urine flowed and her creatinine quickly dropped to a fairly normal level.

Sarah was home in a few days, elated, but heavily immuno-suppressed and vulnerable to opportunistic infections. As most of you already know, the greatest chance for acute rejection of a new kidney is in the first few months. Luckily, this time passed without problems.

Sarah enjoyed several excellent years, with her kidney doing its job and her Lupus seemingly in remission. For those with kidney issues, it can seem like a miracle to have this time of freedom from dialysis and all the other issues. It's easy to write that she 'enjoyed several excellent years', but not as easy to explain what a wonderful time this was for Sarah. Unfortunately, it did come to an end.

When she came to see me a few years later, it was because her calf was swollen and tender. An ultrasound of the lower extremity revealed a clot in a large vein. This is called a deep vein thrombosis, or DVT, potentially very dangerous because a piece of the clot can break off and travel into a large artery in the lungs. This, in turn, is called a pulmonary embolus, which can be life threatening.

A comprehensive blood panel was drawn. Shockingly, it revealed elevated creatinine, setting off what the medical staffs often call a 'Sherlock Holmes' search for the cause of both the thrombosis and abnormal kidney results. Were they related or was this just a coincidence?

It turned out they were related and treatment for both was the same. For reasons unknowable, Sarah had manifested a complication of Lupus not previously seen during her illness. She had developed a peculiar antibody circulating in her blood that causes clotting. It's called an anti-cardiolipin antibody.

She was prescribed treatment to prevent further blood clots, while dissolving existing clots, using intravenous heparin, an anti-coagulant, followed by coumadin, an oral medication that prevents clotting. It was urgent to establish just the right dose of each, to prevent clotting and bleeding. Levels too low could invite clotting. Levels too high could cause spontaneous bleeding.

Sarah was admitted to the hospital where she received intravenous heparin, preventing further clotting while allowing the existing clot to dissolve and be rendered harmless. Small blood vessels that fed Sarah's new kidney had also clotted. Her calf pain improved and the swelling abated as the blood clot dissolved, but she had lost some kidney function due to the small-vessel clots.

Nonetheless, her body proved strong and resilient, in no small part because her spirits remained strong and she chose a positive emotional path. Her kidney lasted 11 healthy, strong years. Then, her body slowly began to show signs that it was rejecting the kidney. However, there was enough forewarning for us to amply prepare for her next kidney transplant. Her aunt, to assure Sarah she would not need to go on dialysis again, volunteered to donate. Sarah was 39 years old when she received transplant number three, from her mother's sister.

Although it was a gift of love, things did not go well from the start. The kidney failed immediately, in fact, due to a rare phenomenon called hyper-acute rejection—a rapid, severe reaction within the new kidney caused by circulating antibodies that immediately attack it. Not only did the kidney never function, it became toxic and Sarah suffered pain and a high fever, even as the kidney was surgically removed.

The moment doctors removed the rejected kidney, Sarah's symptoms abated, but so did her immediate hopes of living a normal life. She was deflated and fell into an emotional depression. Her support group also suffered. Her mother ached for her and her aunt felt like a failure. Her sisters, seeing Sarah so low, were devastated. Everything seemed dark and hopeless. The family struggled against the undertow of grief.

Then, another miracle happened. Sarah's father, who had become chairman of the mathematics department at Indiana University, a consuming and challenging job, nevertheless stepped forward and offered to donate his kidney to his daughter. Sarah and the rest of the family broke down and cried tears of joy for a long time after blood tests indicated that father and daughter were compatible. Her fourth transplant took place in 2009, at Cedars Sinai.

Shortly after the operation, Dr. Cohen, the surgeon who'd performed all of Sarah's transplants, met with her family. In a moment worthy of an Oscar-winning film, he told them the procedure had been a success. Sarah and her father were both find and Sarah's kidney produced urine as soon as it was hooked up. The family, once more broke into tears of joy.

Sarah, living in Santa Barbara, walked on the beaches and breathed deep every day. She was again enjoying the magical benefits of normal kidney function. She saw hope on the horizon, as joyous as the playful dolphins that arced out of the surf, seemingly celebrating with her. Surely, she thought, this would end the nightmarish merry-go-round of anticipation and deflation that had plagued most of her life.

But, more obstacles lay ahead.

During the early course of her fourth transplant, Sarah's platelet count began to drop to a dangerously low level. Platelets are sticky, disc-shaped cells in the blood that the body needs for blood to clot during bleeding. Lupus is notoriously associated with a low platelet count. In Sarah's case, we tracked its cause to an enlarged spleen, which grew bigger over time with her decreasing platelet count. In a sort of Catch-22, an enlarged spleen destroys platelets faster than bone marrow can produce them, which, in turn, causes the spleen to grow even larger. If the platelet count drops below about 20,000 (normal levels are 150,000 to 400,000), the chance of spontaneous bleeding skyrockets.

I was very conscious of the maddening complexity of Sarah's medical challenges. On one hand, her previously functioning kidney was severely damaged by her tendency to clot. On the other hand, her falling platelet count now put her at risk for subsequent bleeding. Meanwhile, her spleen had to be removed—another major operation. Sarah found it hard to even process the notion of another operation, but she had always trusted my judgement, and in the end, she agreed to it. The surgery successfully returned her platelet count to normal.

Sarah had many MRI (Magnetic Resonance Imaging) scans, used as diagnostic tools, during her long, complex medical journey. At the time, gadolinium, a contrast agent thought to be harmless, was employed to enhance MRI images, important for accurate diagnosis. But, when Sarah received her fourth transplant, a few cases were emerging of kidney-disease patients who had undergone several MRI scans with exposure to gadolinium, then developed a peculiar disease called *Nephrogenic Fibrosing Sclerosis* (NFS).

Sarah's kidney functioned well, but she told me she was feeling progressively more uncomfortable. Initially she felt like her skin tingled, a symptom followed by progressive thickening and tightening of her skin, especially in her legs, which ultimately interfered with walking. Her joints ached and she fatigued easily. Blood tests revealed new evidence of generalized inflammation, raising concern that her Lupus was reactivating, yet specific Lupus tests remained unchanged.

During this time, more NFS cases were being diagnosed. After reading an article on the subject, the proverbial 'light bulb' flickered in my mind. I wondered if Sarah be suffering from this newly discovered disease. My first reaction was that fate couldn't be that cruel, but the more I thought about it, I knew it could be the answer.

All I could do is shake my head when NFS was confirmed by a consultant experienced with it. Sarah, who had already been through so much, had developed this horrendous reaction to multiple gadolinium exposures. There was no specific treatment and no knowledge of the course that NFS, a newcomer to the pathology world, would take. Could it destroy her dad's kidney by causing similar thickening in the renal tissue? There was no way to know.

For the next several months, we closely monitored her progress. I increased her steroid dose because of severe inflammatory symptoms related to her NFS. Her aches gradually abated, but her skin continued to harden and it began to feel like wood. The tissue around her legs grew cement-like, making walking extremely difficult. Then, in addition to her NFS-induced symptoms, she began to feel severe pain in her hips. X-rays revealed severe, bone-on-bone arthritis in both hips.

She was struggling on heroically, but I knew something had to be done to improve her quality of her life. Over the next few months, everything went downhill for her. She became almost immobile, riddled with pain when she tried to walk, and was becoming emotionally depleted, losing any semblance of hope. She asked me more than once, "What have I done to deserve this?" I had no answer, but I always followed up her question with quiet and positive statements about her road back to health.

Still, Sarah imagined herself at hell's gate, flames licking at her body. "Every part of me hurts, aches, stings, and burns," she told me. "My life has no value or purpose. Instead of becoming an actor, I've become a lifelong patient. I will never have children or the opportunity for romance. My family has sacrificed everything for me, not only their kidneys, but their lives have been stalled by supporting me throughout my perpetual disease. I love them so much and want so desperately to give back to them. I feel hopeless and feeble. Sometimes I feel death would be a better choice."

When things like this happen to our patients, many doctors have to dig deep to meet the challenge. Hearing patients describe their misery, as Sarah did, can produce profound sadness in those around her, along with feelings of helplessness and of failure. As one of her primary physicians, I had to fight those feelings myself. This 'physician's challenge' is not easy. When we deal with extremely challenged patients, we must bring clinical competence and empathy, because we bear the weight of shepherding a patient successfully through illness. That's why, frankly, so many doctors burn out, or grow a self-protective shell that patients might term a 'poor bedside manner'.

Combining state-of-the-art technical support with empathy requires spending more time with patients, tending to the soul, asking about feelings, listening, and at times seeking support from appropriate specialists to diminish suffering from anxiety, depression, and suicidal thoughts.

The Greek physician Hippocrates, known as the father of modern medicine and famous for his 'oath' for practicing doctors, may have said it best: *"I will remember that there is art to medicine as well as science, and that warmth, sympathy, and understanding may outweigh the surgeon's knife or the chemist's drug."*

Still, the fact remains, sometimes nature takes a course that we may not have chosen. Nature, of course, isn't kind or cruel and doesn't choose sides or pick winners and losers. It is ambivalent and behaves in accordance with the laws of physics, chemistry and biology. It has, essentially, no soul, no conscience and no sense of guilt or equality. We can do much to deal with disease, but it often chooses its own course.

Such was the case for Sarah, for whom every open door was ultimately slammed shut by some new, unexpected, soulless complication. It wasn't the medical system's fault and it sure as hell wasn't her fault. It just "was," and it was our role to make the best of that.

Once again, I designed a credible plan that would bring her some relief and help her regain hope. It wasn't easy, considering her roller-coaster history with hope, and the fact that she'd been dealt so many bad hands. There were, though, some good and fortunate cards dealt to her, as well – her 11-year success with one kidney and the fact that she has had wonderful support from her family – and it was my job to help her focus on those.

Her newest challenge was not a small one. Her forced increased steroid dose to treat NFS, plus her sedentary state, caused weight gain, adding to her immobility. Pain from the severe arthritis in both hips precluded physical therapy and an exercise program that would get her moving, help her lose weight and help prevent cardiovascular disease.

She was down. I remember her, asking me with tears in her eyes, "Is this the best of my fate? I know I'll never have children or become the actor I dreamed of becoming, but am I going to be confined to a wheelchair the rest of my life? What is this new monster inside me going to do?"

I took her hand and pointed out that her father's kidney was still functioning well. That was the primary thing. On that positive note, Sarah and I strategized. I suggested a hip replacement would immediately eliminate much of her arthritic pain. I suggested a minimal-incision approach that would reduce postoperative pain and allow her to walk immediately after surgery. After that, she'd have time to 'train' for a second hip replacement, which we would schedule six months later. Our plan called for Sarah to receive two new hips, start physical therapy, improve her diet, lose weight and resume what she loved most – singing and being with friends.

Her right-hip surgery went well and Sarah enjoyed immediate pain relief. She had the same result with her left hip and we had a small celebration. She was feeling so much better, and after all she had been through, she had no pain! She knew, by then, to take every minute as it came, to enjoy it and not think too far ahead. Life, she knew, was about 'right now'. I have found over the years that the patients who grasp this crucial concept are often those who stay the healthiest.

For Sarah, the next few years sailed by uneventfully in terms of medical nightmares. She still faced a number of health issues and she often had to drag her weary self to Pilates to gain strength and flexibility, not easy for a body ravaged by Lupus, steroid toxicity and NFS, let alone dialysis and four kidney transplants. But, then again, this was Sarah, and her dogged pursuit of wellness remained undiminished. Finally, she felt well enough to dare to fulfill one of her dreams – to visit Paris. And that, of course, is where we came into this story. With Big Ed at her side, Sarah set off for France and a dream. She felt she could literally fly without the plane, she was so excited. Her flight was uneventful, unfortunately, her visit to the City of Light would not be.

An attendant met Sarah at the airport, wheeling her through customs and the baggage claim. A friend met her at the airport and they wedged Sarah, her baggage, and Big Ed into a car and drove to Sarah's hotel. For the first few hours, she felt as wonderful and wandered the boulevards, smiling the entire time. Sarah's entire first week in France was magical—lunch at the top of the Eiffel Tower and tours of the Louvre and Notre Dame. She felt happy and carefree for the first time she could remember.

Then, I got a phone call at three o'clock in the morning. I hadn't taken calls for a while, but I remember getting an instant uneasy feeling in my stomach. I quickly grabbed the phone. I said, "Hello," and then I heard Sarah crying. I knew she was in France and I knew something was terribly wrong. Finally, in a small, trembling voice, she told me she had been out walking along a Paris street when she stumbled and fell. She was still there, on the sidewalk. Responding to my questions, she said she didn't think she had broken any bones, but she felt very sick and her hips hurt badly and her pain was increasing. She said she was on a small side street and there were no taxis, but she thought she could walk, and she wasn't far from her hotel. It was late morning in Paris and I told her, in a calm voice, to walk back, if she could, and have the hotel concierge find ice to put on her injury. Then she should have the concierge help her find a hospital emergency room where a physician could evaluate her. I reminded her to tell the medical staff that she was taking a blood thinner and that she might be bleeding internally.

I made sure that when Sarah left for Paris, her INR (International

Normalized Ratio, a system for reporting the results of blood clotting tests) was in its usual therapeutic range. She had been taking the same blood thinner for years to prevent the clotting syndrome caused by Lupus.

Still, I was very worried.

Sarah told me as she walked back to her hotel – I made sure she stayed on the line the entire time – that she didn't see any swelling. She hung up when she got back to the hotel, which as it turned out, was unfortunate because the ice relieved her pain so she didn't visit the ER. I would have strongly advised the visit and I hung up only because she said she was going to. In hindsight that was a mistake, though understandable for a person who hadn't known wellness in years and didn't care much for hospitals.

Early the next morning, I called her and our conversation was quite different. She sounded terrified. Her thigh was badly swollen and her pain severe. A friend she knew is Paris drove her to the ER of an excellent French hospital, where a diagnosis revealed active bleeding inside her thigh. Her red blood cell count was dangerously low, her INR was dangerously elevated, (suggesting presence of too much blood thinner). Her blood pressure was extremely low, so low it could damage her kidney for lack of adequate blood supply. Worst of all, her creatinine level had climbed to 3.8, signaling a critical, acute renal injury.

For all her previous challenges, the following weeks were among Sarah's most harrowing. Blood transfusions boosted blood volume and pressure. Vitamin K normalized her INR, allowing the huge hematoma in her soft tissue to slowly regress. Still, she remained in a medical "Twilight Zone," in a foreign country. She was terrified. She was given opiates to help reduce the pain, but they played havoc with her ability to think clearly or communicate in French. Dopey, confused, a stranger in a strange land, she just wanted to go home. But, she was far too sick. Deeply concerned, as we all were, her father flew to Paris and remained with Sarah for the two weeks it took her to stabilize her. What we would learn later was that despite French nephrologists' best efforts, her kidney was irreversibly damaged.

She was so thankful to be back in California, at home, she cried all afternoon. We immediately began medical treatment. Uremic, Sarah quickly required dialysis, but a number of technical problems made that difficult. First, Sarah had used up many vascular sites on her body for previous treatments. She had also clotted off some potential access sites due to her unusual clotting syndrome. I spoke with Sarah and her nephrologists daily, helping her understand they were superb physicians.

Sarah arrived home safely from her ordeal. She required several days in Cottage Hospital to successfully modify her access into one that would function for the long term. It took weeks of dialysis treatment, physical therapy and support from our entire renal team for Sarah to adjust back to dialysis.

It seemed amazing to me that Sarah not only went back on dialysis after years of 'normal' living with several transplants, but she regained a strong, positive attitude about life. Her mother feel victim to a stroke and Sarah found their roles were reversed as she cared for her mother and tried to help her stay strong, as her mother had done for her so many times.

Sometimes, Sarah admitted to me that things did get overwhelming and she did howl in anguish and curse dialysis, but she only did it when she was alone now. It helped her to stay upbeat for her mother.

I worked with Sarah, helping her focus on getting stronger, leaner and healthier, to increase her chances for another kidney. I told her about research on a bio-mechanical kidney in San Francisco and gave her the website to check out. I did not hear from her for several weeks and I considered that a good sign. We met accidentally, though, not long ago. I was finishing an appointment with my dental hygienist (preventative care is essential!) and I heard a voice call out, "Hello Dr. Fisher!"

It was Sarah, she looked fit and her spirits seemed high. We shared a long hug. She said she didn't want a human kidney anymore, but the mechanical one instead. "To be ready, I'm exercising and only eating a healthy, low sugar, low calorie diet."

She was so proud and so was I. Sarah's story is far from over, I believe and I think there are many great parts yet to come. She is an ultimate warrior, a lover of life, and one of the most inspiring, courageous people I've met in 40 years of medical practice. She has beaten the most intim-idating odds. She told me she's even thinking about taking Big Ed on another trip, a shorter one. Her spirit is indomitable. I am truly humbled by her story.

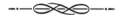

Chapter 4

Mick

Mick stood excited on the edge of the passenger dive-boat. He checked his mask, snorkel, and 17-pound weight belt, adjusted his wet-suit, then took one large step off the vessel and dropped 10 feet into the sea at Anacapa Island, 12 miles off the Ventura, California coast.

Bobbing up like a cork, he gave the "okay" signal to the dive-boat crew, then snorkeled toward the island, 200 yards off. He had no SCU-BA gear. Instead, he preferred to "skin dive," or "breath-hold dive," as some call it.

As Mick snorkeled, he heard gulls, cormorants, and sea lions squawking and barking morning greetings. Once he got to a water depth of 20 feet, he took a deep breath, pointed his face toward the seafloor, his fins toward the sky, and "penciled" his way toward the bot-tom. Fifteen feet down, he swiveled to a horizontal plane and snaked his way through resplendent kelp beds, their broad leaves heaving in a gentle current. The kelp forest was alive with fish, sea urchins, aba-lone, and barnacled rocks of every imaginable color. Bars of morning sunlight barreled through the kelp in broad bands, sparkling like dia-monds off every surface they touched.

After nearly a minute under water, Mick looked to the sea surface, found a good hole in the kelp and popped up, breathing hard, but as alive as he'd ever felt, at one with nature's magical kingdom.

Mick repeated his descents for nearly an hour, then realized he'd better head back to the boat. He was the last to board, receiving a disciplinary wink from the skipper. They knew. Mick was always last returning to the boat. But they also knew he was safe, and they knew what he knew—Mick was good at this, and he was addicted to it.

Back on deck, his wetsuit drawn down around his waist, Mick looked surprisingly lean and muscular, the result of relentless swimming, diving, hiking, and eating healthy food.

Harbor Master for the City of Santa Barbara, Mick is married to his beautiful wife Ginger, loving parents of their college-age son, Cole. He, of all people, knows the importance of finding balance between work, family, exercise, nutrition, and love. Those who know Mick admire him for his intelligence, kindness, wit, patience, ethics, competence, courage and joie de vivre—all of which have rewarded him with a loving family and a terrific job in a beautiful city.

Any casual observer watching Mick work out, looking so fit, even at the age of 68 would be happy to have traveled a similar path with similar results. Those perceptions, however, are but a piece of his story.

If I told you that Mick has spent three years of his life on dialysis, you might find that surprising. Even more astounding is that Mick received four kidney transplants over the past 36 years. In June, 2013, he had his final dialysis treatment at the Santa Barbara Artificial Kidney Center before heading to Cedars Sinai for his fourth transplant.

He was discharged five days later with another new, functioning kidney. He felt better immediately as the organ efficiently filtered waste products from his body, correcting his fluid and electrolyte imbalances. Mick's spirit soared (again) as he sat in a wheelchair, and waved goodbye to nurses who had expertly and kindly attended to him during his recovery.

(The day before his departure, Mick managed to push his intravenous "tree," hung with various lines, drainage bags and such, a half-mile through the corridors of his recovery ward. Asked by a doctor what he was doing, he said, only half-joking, "training for my next transplant.") Ginger's smile and relaxed brow greeted Mick at their car. Her relief and gratitude for the anonymous donor who'd come forward to participate in a paired kidney exchange, mirrored in her tear-filled eyes. (A paired exchange, also known as a "kidney swap" occurs when a living kidney donor is incompatible with their recipient, and so exchanges kidneys with another donor/recipient pair. We'll discuss this more in the next chapter.) Ginger herself, had endured the voyage with Mick, soldiering through the helplessness, fear, and anxiety that grip any caregiver struggling to support a loved one while maintaining a sense of self and an independent identity.

The weight of a long, life-sustaining voyage on dialysis might, just might, be over—again. As he slowly rose from his wheelchair, Mick felt pain at the operative site, weakness in his arms and legs, aching in his joints. In his inimitable style, he declined help, got up slowly, crawled into the passenger seat and off they went, back to Santa Barbara.

Turning the first corner, Mick saw a man smoking a cigarette and just shook his head. "Don't they get it?" he rhetorically asked his wife. "Don't they understand that life, unadulterated by excessive food, drink, or smoking, is God's greatest gift? I understand you might not be able to lengthen your life, but why shorten it?"

Mick enjoyed a renewed sense of hope that day, in part due to what we know about complex immunologic problems that can affect longevity of a new kidney—vastly improved since 1979, when Mick started dialysis, or 1980 when he received his first transplant.

"Dialysis, in the comprehensive sense, was really only 20 years old in 1979," Mick recalls. "The machines looked like Maytag washers and the process of clearing toxic waste was far more punishing and uncontrolled than today. Patients routinely passed out from crashing blood pressure, snapped into agonizing cramps without notice, or, in a few cases, died from poorly managed or inadvertently toxic treatments. It was scary stuff."

Mick vividly remembers dialysis days that interrupted his life several times between 1979 and 2013. Dependence, despair, fleeting suicidal notions, and the sickening feeling of losing freedom continually haunted him.

Through his 36-year dance with kidney disease, however, he always overcame self-pity, for his own wellbeing and because he knew self-pity destroys everything around it. At each challenging juncture, he eventually snapped out of his funk, crafted a plan for escaping dialysis and getting another transplant. "I won't lie," he says. "It takes confidence, hope, guts, self-reliance, even your own medical research, to pull yourself out of a hole like that."

Back aboard the dive-boat, Mick's eyes sprung open, freeing himself from dark visions of the past. He smiled broadly, spontaneously, enjoying his latest jailbreak from the shackles of dialysis life.

After previous kidney transplants, Mick celebrated his revitalized body and spirit in other ways, like competing in racquetball at the U.S. Transplant Games, a multi-sport, Olympic-style competition among transplant athletes of every sort—heart, lung, kidney, liver, pancreas, you name it.

"I remember a doubles final in Salt Lake City," he says. "My lung-transplant buddy Ken and I beat a liver-and-heart duo to win the gold. It was epic. The whole Transplant Games experience was a celebration of life like none other. Thousands of transplant athletes and donor families attended. Ginger even told me on the airplane flight home one time, 'I hope heaven is like the Transplant Games.'"

After a few transplants, you learn to live in the moment and Mick was no exception. He always maintained a strong sense of reality and awareness of "known unknowns" lurking in the shadows. After each new transplant, he still felt anxious awaiting lab-test results. Any slight change in kidney function or a trace of protein in his urine raised the possibility of rejection, though there were always other potential causes ranging from opportunistic infections swarming his immunocompromised body, technical problems from surgery, drug reactions or even erroneous lab results.

Even when a kidney functioned well, Mick lived in a modest state of alert and subliminal fear of something going haywire. It had before, and he knew it could again. A transplant's longevity is never certain. That's why, even several years out with a new kidney, patients like Mick never go more than three months without bloodwork and urinalysis.

Many transplant patients have experienced post-transplant infections, especially in the 1980s and 1990s, when early-rejection episodes were more frequent. Typically, they received high-dose intravenous corticosteroids to reverse the problem. Unfortunately, this treatment also weakened their immune systems and exposure to infections—fungal, bacterial, viral—that often led to hospitalizations, kidney biopsies, imaging studies, and dose-manipulation of immunosuppressant drugs. Back then, getting a kidney to "stick" could be quite a roller-coaster ride. Generally, the ride is smoother today, though vigilant monitoring remains essential.

Those phantoms appeared in different forms during each of Mick's transplants, robbing him of a full sense of stability and certainty. Even during periods of successful transplant, despite roadblocks that inevitably emerged, his motto has been to live life fully, a day at a time.

Sitting on that dive boat, enjoying the stunning island scenery, Mick again grew reflective, climbing aboard the "way-back machine" to his freshman year at UC Santa Barbara, when he first encountered kidney disease and began his circuitous medical odyssey.

New students at UCSB were required to have a physical exam and blood test. A technician drew three vials of blood and obtained a urine sample. At the time, Mick could cared less, his mind wandering between course work, social events, and the Vietnam War, his protest of which ultimately earned him a short stint in state prison. But that's another story (and adversity overcome).

He had no reason to suspect lab results wouldn't be perfect. His family history indicated nothing genetically concerning, and longevity was common, many relatives living into their mid-90s.

The university doctor reviewed the results and told Mick they were perfectly normal, other than a trace of protein in his urine. Mick looks back and remembers those words, "A trace of protein in your urine," noting, "That's the day it all started."

To be safe, Mick followed the doctor's advice to get an x-ray of his kidneys to better visualize their structure and rule out any abnormalities. Then he got the results. The radiologist said Mick had what looked like medullary sponge kidney, a relatively benign birth defect that wouldn't lead to kidney failure. The doctor told him, "Don't worry.

You'll live to be 90, just like your relatives."

Well, Mick might make it to 90 all right, but not via the normal path. Mick graduated from UCSB, eager to enter life's arena, unaware that he was silently losing kidney function and someday he would face full-blown kidney failure. The hurricane hit seven years later. A commercial fisherman at the time, Mick was at sea one day when he began feeling listless, and, he says, "A sort of weird kind of sick," He also had an unquenchable thirst. Drinking more water, he thought, was simply a healthy way to live. But he was visibly pale, losing appetite and sleeping poorly. His ankles were swollen. Something was wrong.

His internist sat Mick down to discuss the results of his laboratory tests. "These are so out of whack, your blood must have coagulated in the tube," he said. "Let's repeat the test." The second results were no better. "Your kidneys have failed," he reported, with a fearful tone. "You need immediate dialysis, or you may die very soon." Thankfully, the physician's office was across the street from Cottage Hospital, where Mick was immediately admitted for emergency dialysis.

At the time, I was a new nephrologist in Santa Barbara, fresh from my internal medicine and nephrology training at UCLA. My practice was growing, but up until I consulted on Mick, I'd mostly seen older patients who were more likely to have chronic kidney disease. When I initially saw Mick, I was shocked. He was barely younger than I, and because it was so easy to identify with him, I internalized his fear and anxiety. I realized right then that only chance separated us. Words of a Joan Baez song, "There but for fortune go you or I," played in my mind's ear. My heart went out to him.

"I remember meeting Dr. Fisher the first time," Mick recalls. "Young, handsome and, I could tell immediately, warm of heart and spirit. After our consultation, he said, 'We're going to make you well. We're going to get you a kidney transplant if that's what it takes.' Those few words, the hope and determination, changed my life forever."

Mick needed immediate dialysis to reverse perilous effects of a very high serum potassium level and severe metabolic acidosis. In addition, it would remove extra fluid—15 pounds of it—he'd retained as his kidneys failed. Mick appeared confused, but he understood the need for urgent treatment. I promised him dialysis would make him feel better. A vascular surgeon placed a shunt just above Mick's right ankle, one end in a vein, the other in an artery.

Ultrasound imaging of his kidneys revealed sad news—they were small, consistent with chronic nephritis, an inflammation of the kidneys possibly resulting from a childhood streptococcus ("Strep") infection that led to slow, unrelenting immunologic damage to his kidneys (see post-infectious glomerulonephritis in Chapter 2).

During his first week in the hospital, Mick received daily dialysis. As his mind cleared and uremia symptoms abated, I explained to him that there was no treatment to restore his kidney function, and that he would need ongoing dialysis to maintain his health. Grasping for stoicism, he winced visibly at the disturbing news.

During one of Mick's early treatments I learned that he had an older brother who lived on the east coast. I immediately envisioned a living-related transplant—Mick's best chance for a normal life. As we spoke of the possibilities, hope slowly supplanted sadness and despair, and for the first time I saw more smiles than not. To see Mick light up that way lifted my spirits as well. After our conversations about transplantation, Mick grew more determined.

"I know now I won't spend a lifetime on dialysis," he told me. "I just won't."

Mick's turnabout from grief to determination proved an epiphany for me that would influence the way I approached patients throughout my medical career. Offer hope and possibility, but never false hope. Provide positive sentiment early on, when the patient needs it the most. Discharged from the hospital, Mick started a three-day-a-week dialysis regimen. He initially felt better, had more energy, and began to enjoy food (he also said he had far more dates—an unexpected side effect of losing weight, getting color back, and feeling well). We talked about starting an exercise program and pursuing a transplant.

His mood was steady and upbeat as we worked to fine-tune his health and ready him for the next step. He fit perfectly into the "honeymoon period" described by Norman B Levy MD in his book "Living or Dying," which describes patients' early sense of exhilaration, the relief of well-being as they recover from a uremic state.

But Mick's honeymoon period ended abruptly.

He had befriended a lady in her seventies, Betty Glazer, who sat in a dialysis chair next to him. She was intelligent, gracious, and had been receiving treatments for about eighteen months. She had been a first-grade teacher, but now her greatest pleasure came from her grandchildren and her loving husband of forty-five years. She willingly and gratefully accepted dialysis treatments because to her, life at almost any cost was precious.

Betty and Mick discussed their situations, shared their feelings, and talked philosophy. Mick grew very fond of her, admiring her spunk and spirit. Unfortunately, Betty also had diabetes and coronary artery disease. Recently she had experienced shortness of breath and was scheduled to see a cardiologist.

On a Wednesday morning Mrs. Glazer came in for her routine treatment, which began with a problem. Suddenly, she clutched her chest and her machine "alarmed," signaling a blood-pressure drop. Nurses rushed to her and found her without a pulse. Despite quick application of CPR, and, though curtained off, Mick had seen enough to know his friend had died. Nausea squeezed his stomach, his heart raced, and perspiration beaded his forehead.

At that moment, Mick knew he had to talk to his brother. He desperately needed rescue from this nightmare that would certainly end poorly. That night he called Tony.

"When I learned that my brother Mick had come back sick from a fishing trip—I mean, sick, in a life-threatening way—I was shocked and scared," Tony recalls. "Mick's professional life exposed him to all sorts of dangers, but I never imagined he would be in mortal danger from a cause I couldn't have guessed and didn't understand. I just assumed that he and I would live forever; I suppose deep down I still do. Anyway, Mick called me in Connecticut, where I lived, and we had a long talk about dialysis and his future. I don't remember whether it was in that first call or a later one that Mick raised the question of whether I would consider being a kidney donor. As I recall, I said something noncommittal, and told Mick I would talk to my doctors.

"Then the roof fell in. My wife and I separated, and I spiraled into a state of emotional exhaustion. I told Mick I couldn't deal with anything else for the time being. I think he understood but felt wounded by my disregard for him. Things kind of simmered along for a few months. Mick and I weren't exactly estranged, but I would say our relationship was strained.

"I was young and preoccupied with my own life, paying less attention to my brother's pain than my own. Then the clouds began to clear. I realized that my life wasn't over. I couldn't know it then, but it was only just beginning. And I realized that I needed and wanted to do what I could for Mick—the only brother I'd ever have.

"I came back to the question of donating a kidney and decided to pursue it in earnest. None of the doctors I spoke to seemed terribly concerned about the risks. I was in good health, and they saw no reason I shouldn't go ahead . . . if I wanted. So, the ball was back in my court. When someone (I don't remember who) told me that insurance companies don't distinguish between people with one kidney and those with two so far as life insurance policies are concerned, I thought, 'Well, isn't it ridiculous I've waited so long?'

So, I decided to do it, and called Mick to let him know. The rift immediately healed on both sides. I wasn't frightened, and in fact didn't even really think about what lay ahead until I checked into the hospital for the operation. Then and afterward, people said to me, 'how generous, how brave, etc.' None of that ever made any sense to me. I was helping my brother, as most people would, and the risks were so minimal that if being a donor counted as bravery, I would say the price of admission was getting credit on the cheap. The only real cost was a few days of discomfort (the worst being a catheter they removed with a yank).

I was back in the pool swimming ten days after the operation and haven't stopped since. When I think back on those days, I have a good feeling about it all, especially about my brother, for whom my love gets deeper every year. I know I did a good thing—I wouldn't elevate it beyond that—but it's given me a long afterlife of pleasure that was worth ten thousand times the price of admission."

In 1980, there existed little long-term data on safety for a kidney donor, as transplants themselves were relatively new. In addition, laparoscopic kidney removal, the modern-day alternative to the painful, open surgery Tony endured, didn't exist at the time. Tony was also under great emotional duress when Mick fell ill. Once he made up his mind, however, his pivot to save his brother was swift and his courage to face any potential danger steadfast. He acted purely out of brotherly love. That's what heroes do. They don't throw touchdown passes. They donate kidneys.

Following successful transplant surgery at UCLA, Mick went from agony to ecstasy and began to live a full, rich life. He had excellent kidney function and was on low-dose immuno-suppressants. We lost contact for intermittent periods, during which important testing didn't get done. In hindsight, we were both too complacent because of his perfect function.

In March,1993, Mick excitedly told me that he and Ginger were getting married. He made an appointment for a physical exam and a blood-draw, simple requirements for his marriage license. Stunned, I saw abnormal results indicating kidney failure. I ached for Mick and Ginger, who had no idea what they faced to start their marriage.

"I remember sitting in Dr. Fisher's office, tears streaming down his cheeks," Mick recalls. "He seemed equally devastated as me. We looked at each other with that 'Oh my God, what now?' kind of expression. Immediately, however, he jumped into action."

Mick's kidney was swollen because the ureter that allowed urine to drain into the bladder was swollen, secondary to rejection. We placed a stent into the ureter to allow drainage and increased his immuno-suppressants. Despite all efforts, however, Mick's kidney function continued declining at an alarming rate.

Mick was planning to start law school and Ginger was going to pursue a degree in communications after they married in June. They had already planned a honeymoon in Italy. I recommended cancelling it because Mick would likely need dialysis sooner rather than later. The wedding was on, but the honeymoon was put on hold.

Devastated but resilient, they settled on a getaway in San Francisco. "Between March, when I felt well and had my blood test, and June, when we got married, I grew so terribly ill I could barely make it through the ceremony." Mick says. "I remember going to a baseball game in Oakland, but everything on that makeshift honeymoon was a struggle. I was back in hell."

Ginger says her "world had grown gloomy and small." She received great support from family and friends, but seeing her husband growing more ill by the day, she made a monumental decision to donate a kidney to him. Very few unrelated living transplants had been performed, but Mick saw through initial resistance to this "new" approach, which he now describes, with palpable frustration, as 'moral and ethical cowardice.'

"At the time, I knew the notion of living, non-related transplants seemed foreign to American medicine, and that made no sense to me," he recalls. "I mean, if you can receive a working kidney from a dead person, why couldn't a living, non-related person donate, probably with equal or better results?"

So, Mick settled on a plan.

"I traveled to Los Angeles, where I spent a week at my mother's house. Each day, I went to the UCLA Medical Library. I combed the stacks, looking for articles about living, non-related transplants. And then I found it—a study from Brazil reviewing results from 2,200 patients who received living, non-related transplants. Outcomes were excellent, on a par with or exceeding those from cadaveric transplants. My research also revealed that in the U.S., reticence to perform these surgeries was borne of an ethical, not medical, concern, that is, a fear that living, non-related transplants would lead to a market in human organs. Silly, even ridiculous, in hindsight."

Cedars Sinai was excited to perform a living, nonrelated transplant between Mick and Ginger—the 13th they'd done in this new, enlightened era (they've done thousands since). Genetic testing showed good compatibility, and they cleared Ginger and Mick for transplant. "When we got the results, we rolled around on the carpet, hugging and crying, again buoyed by the possibility of life restored," Mick remembers.

Cedars admitted Mick and Ginger on September 14, 1993—on separate floors. On their gurneys beside each other, wheeling toward separate operating rooms the next day, Mick said, "Please stop, I want to kiss my wife." Orderlies pushed their gurneys together. Pressing his lips to

Ginger's, he whispered, "I love you, sweetheart. You're my hero." Ginger recalls nurses crying at the sight.

Two days later, Ginger's mother wheeled her through the hospital corridor to see her husband for the first time. They just held hands, laughed and cried. "We did it," Mick managed to croak in between tears, Ginger nodded vigorously through her own sobs of joy, like she would three years later, in labor giving birth to their son, Cole.

The successful transplant also put Mick and Ginger in the news, the last place they expected to land. Turns out that theirs was only the 100th spousal transplant in the country at the time. Press interviews, an article in *Ladies Home Journal*, a talk show called "Northwest Afternoon" in Seattle—it came like an avalanche.

Mick told a local newspaper reporter, "Health is a precious gift and love really does heal. People who donate kidneys are the true heroes of the nineties." In the *Ladies Home Journal* article, Ginger said, "I don't feel heroic; I just did what I knew had to be done for the man I love. I think of my donation as a special bond we'll share the rest of our lives."

The emotional yo-yo quietly spun down and Ginger returned to work in three weeks, rejoining aerobic classes soon after. Six months following the transplant, Mick was back playing racquetball and swimming. In May 1994, Mick and Ginger made good on their postponed honeymoon to Italy.

I wish the story ended with Ginger's gift to Mick, but this is real life, not reality television. When Cole came along, he was the love of their lives, a miracle child who brought Mick and Ginger the happiness only parents can know. Mick decided against law school, instead following a career in journalism.

This lovely vision played out until one day, 12 years post-transplant, a urinalysis showed traces of protein. Chronic rejection due to recurring glomerulonephritis in his new kidney was back, confirmed via biopsy.

Once again, Mick, Ginger, and I felt the nausea.

Attuned to his body, Mick felt the steady loss of function. When the slightest anemia of renal disease appeared, he knew it. Mick swam to stay in shape, but his lap-times progressively slowed. He saw foamy urine and suspected protein loss. He felt jittery and knew his blood pressure was up.

Before a needle ever punctured his vein for a blood draw, Mick knew he was in trouble again. In fact, he called me, suspecting the worst. And tests confirmed the worst.

Back on the merry-go-round.

While grieving the impending loss of her/his kidney, Mick and Ginger remained laser-focused on the future, thinking about where he could get his next transplant. Mick shared his proactive approach with other dialysis patients. He believed there were altruistic potential donors who would gladly donate a kidney to a friend or a loved one if they were better informed, if they only knew the patient needed one. (Mick displayed considerable empathy for Latino patients from lower socio-economic backgrounds, of whom there was a burgeoning number, and for whom English was often a second language. Many of them had no understanding of how to navigate the medical system and gain access to a transplant. He's spoken with me often about educating this under-served population.)

Mick turned to social media to get the word out. Emails flew to hundreds of loved ones, friends, colleagues, church members, and more. The City Administrator for whom he worked at the City of Santa Barbara even sent an email "blast" to 1,100 employees, explaining Mick's plight and opportunities to help him.

Finally, Dana McCorkle, son of a fisherman friend, stepped forward to donate. When Mick asked him why he would do such a kind thing, Dana said, "You and my father go back 30 years. I want to see you grow old together."

Other potential donors offered too, but Dana was the best genetic match. At a meeting during preoperative testing at Cedars Sinai, a nurse Mick knew well concluded her PowerPoint presentation to prospective donors and recipients, then turned to him and asked, "Mick, did I leave anything out?"

"Well, actually, yes, one thing," he replied. "Keep countertops and kitchenware clean and sanitary. Set your dishwasher on high-heat. The last thing you need is a food-borne illness." The nurse smiled and thanked him. By now, this health-care team was family.

In October 2007, Mick was back in business with a new kidney—his third transplant, magically, delicately placed in his abdomen by the hands of renown, world-class surgeon, Dr. Louis Cohen.

But challenges still lay ahead. After a patient receives several transplants, a process of immunological "sensitization" occurs. This means that with so much foreign tissue in the recipient's body, the immune system responds with antibodies that circulate and eventually harm the new organ—a fact that played a large part in his chronic rejection of Ginger's kidney.

Mick settled back into life after the transplant, working as the Harbor Master, a teenager's dad, a wife's husband. By now, he had set aside his journalism career, during which he published 1,500 magazine articles and earned a prestigious literary award. How he accomplished all this amid periodic health crises is hard to comprehend, but it speaks to creativity, tenacity, and talent. After his third transplant, in fact, he wrote a popular book on Santa Barbara's commercial fishing history. And of course, he continued to swim, hike and lift weights.

"It's pretty straightforward," he says. "If you've got the gift of life, use it. Honor that life, honor the gift, honor the giver."

During the time frame of this kidney transplant, Mick experienced several severe episodes of an intestinal infection caused by a bacterium called *clostridium difficile*. It's a normal organism, part of the flora in the human intestine, but if a patient receives frequent antibiotics, the organism may overgrow, leading to severe diarrhea and vomiting. It thrives, as well, in immuno-suppressed individuals like Mick.

When Mick had bouts of this infection, colloquially known as "C-diff," he grew dehydrated, which elevated his BUN and creatinine. After hydration, they returned to normal, but every episode frightened him. One time, in the hospital with C-diff, Mick looked up at me, exhausted from a vomiting spell, and asked, "Is this just another bump in road?"

"Yes," I replied. "Just a bump in the road."

Three years after his third kidney transplant, Mick again began spilling protein in his urine. A biopsy showed the chronic rejection seen in patients highly sensitized from previous transplants. Mick was not too surprised at the results because he had been through the same process two times before. Still, the sting of the results burrowed in, deep and painful.

The cumulative emotional and physical insults caused by years of recurrent renal failure, dialysis, hospitalizations, renal transplants, anxiety, depression, and pain hammered Mick and Ginger.

With consultation from Cedars' transplant team, we undertook a vigorous attempt to reverse the rejection. Despite frequent plasmapheresis treatments to remove harmful antibodies, plus infusion of immuno-suppressant drugs, his creatinine level steadily rose. Mick's spirits went the opposite direction. Realizing he would require dialysis soon, he struggled with depression—really the first time he was physically and emotionally enervated since his initial encounter with kidney failure. Ginger was very frightened because Mick seemed helpless. She began to despair, thinking he might die.

Weak, confused, sleep-deprived, and emotionally frail, Mick needed help. I knew the only way to reverse this situation was a full-court press, providing both physical and emotional respite. Ginger, drained from years of battling kidney disease alongside Mick, felt equally vulnerable to depression and desperation. She needed tremendous support to overcome this new, potentially catastrophic, situation. Luckily, she had reserves—a wellspring of inner strength absorbed from friends, plus regular visits to Hospice for comfort and emotional guidance.

Finally, Mick headed back to dialysis, back on the medical conveyor belt, less confident of his future than ever. But he sure hadn't lost his pluck. "Even when I returned to dialysis," he says, "in the care of wonderful nurses, I kept telling them, 'You know I'm not staying here, you know that, right?'"

Mick remembers clearly his return to dialysis. "When I was bored and feeling blue, I sat in my chair, watching my blood circulating and I thought about how many ways I could kill myself to make it look like an accident, so my family could receive life-insurance benefits." Fleeting thoughts, thankfully, that he never intended to indulge. After all, he couldn't leave Ginger and Cole behind. "Most of the time, I just kept my head down, reading during treatments," he says. "I didn't care to look around at all the despair. The good news? I finished a lot of books, including Moby Dick—arguably the greatest American novel."

Finally, though, Mick needed anti-depressive medication to improve his mood, help him sleep better, and enjoy his food. Now, we could discuss his future. I could see a renewed spark as he contemplated possibilities.

Mick returned to work as Harbor Master, a demanding job that requires supervising a large staff, dealing with legal and political issues, making difficult decisions, and working with the boating public. He would arrive late for dialysis, harried and exhausted from work, no time to catch his breath, talk to his family, or decompress. "When I left work for dialysis, I remember telling colleagues, with the best smile I could muster, 'See you tomorrow, I'm going to get squeezed.'"

Meanwhile, Mick's indomitable spirit remained. One evening, after dialysis and a long, solo walk, he came into his house, gently held Ginger's face and pointed into his own eyes. "I'm still in here, darling. I swear to you I'm still in here."

At 8:00 pm on May 17, 2013, Mick slumped toward his car following a monthly Harbor Commission meeting, thinking, "Thank God, I made it through another one." At the car, he found messages on three phones—home, cell, and work. Cedars Sinai had a donor for him—an anonymous Good Samaritan who simply wanted to make somebody well. She'd been in Cedars' donor pool for some time and was an excellent match for Mick.

The night passed slowly. Mick could hardly wait to speak with nurses the next morning. When he did, they told him they wanted to move fast and "get (him) on the table within a month." After 22 months on dialysis and some whirlwind pre-testing, Mick got his fourth kidney transplant on June 14, 2013, a paired exchange that included his angel donor and a friend from work who offered Mick a kidney that proved incompatible but matched another recipient well.

"When I needed a fourth transplant, several potential donors stepped up to help," Mick says. "I actually developed a plan to increase my odds of success. The way I figured it, the more donors who got evaluated, the more potential—I hate to put it this way—for "trade bait" in a paired exchange. This is exactly what transpired in the end. The double-surgeries included a friend of mine from work (who learned about my situation from the City Administrator's email) and turned out to be Cedars' first paired exchange."

Two years later, Mick was training to swim to San Francisco from Alcatraz. He was in tip-top shape but unfortunately, became ill with a nasty viral infection just a few weeks before the swim. It took Mick a long time to recover from the body aches and malaise that accompanied it. Though disappointed to have missed the Alcatraz swim, he went back to training for ocean free-diving. To this day, he dives deep below the ocean surface to see how long he can hold his breath before coming up for air. He swims four miles a week, lifts weights, and hikes with his wife.

Mick continues serving Santa Barbara as Harbor Master, while he and Ginger prepare to celebrate their 25th wedding anniversary. Cole will soon graduate from UC Santa Cruz. Mick's new kidney, nearly five years in its new home, functions well, and besides an occasional squamous cell cancer of the skin, his health remains excellent.

So, the dance continues, but for now Mick leads and kidney disease sits on the sidelines.

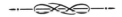

Chapter 5

Mary

In March 2007, Mary's life was in high gear. She was 44 years old, married, with a beautiful 10-year-old daughter. Her Santa Barbara practice as a marriage and family therapist was thriving. She was fit and attractive. Her life wasn't perfect, of course, but every day seemed to hold promise that something good would happen. She had no idea she was on a collision course with a locomotive of ill-health rumbling straight at her.

Mary wrote about the aftermath of that collision and has graciously allowed me to capture some of her account here. If you believe in silver linings, and I do, there are more than one in this story. Primary among them is how Mary, who plummeted into despairing darkness over a period of years, has revitalized and found deep, fulfilling meaning in her life.

She still dialyzes three times a week, but her resolve is strong, and she continues to pursue her dreams. For example, Mary's battle with her oncoming disease motivated her to earnestly take up writing. Despite all she's been through, she recently wrote and published her first book, which, interestingly, is not about her medical challenges, but a call for the country to come together to heal its own political and cultural wounds. *Saving America's Grace*, is a fine book, a perfect example of what people can accomplish, even when fighting chronic disease—in this case, complete renal failure. As Mary has shown, life can blossom, you can triumph over the roughest terrain. But, let me get out of the way, and let Mary tell her story in her own words.

"I remember the first hint that something was wrong. I was attending a personal growth workshop and I started shifting around in my chair, trying to get comfortable. 'Damn, these jeans are getting tight,' I thought to myself. I laughed, thinking maybe I should change my focus from procrastination to weight loss.

"During the next couple of weeks, humor dissipated as, to my confusion and then shock, my ankles grew increasingly swollen. Day by day, they got so huge there was no definition between my foot and calf. In street vernacular, I had 'cankels.' I pointed it out to colleagues and joked about having elephantiasis. Though maybe a tad culturally insensitive, it was funny. Until it wasn't. No doubt, many of you reading this can relate to that feeling."

"I had no idea what was wrong, and tried to ignore it, thinking I was allergic to something and it would soon go away. Then, one day in early spring, I took my daughter to see a pediatrician. I was wearing shorts and when the pediatrician saw my swollen ankles, she showed serious concern. 'You are the one who needs to see a doctor,' she said, with enough urgency to frighten me. I immediately visited my internist, who put me through a series of tests, results of which turned my life upside down."

A urinalysis revealed that Mary's kidneys were leaking 4.5 grams of protein a day, which dismayed her doctors because a normal amount is about 40 times less. Her tests also showed she also had extremely high cholesterol.

"I couldn't believe it because I had no idea what 'leaking protein' meant and I had never had high cholesterol before," she said. "I was always careful about my health. I worked out, watched what I ate, and saw my doctor regularly. It was hard to believe what was happening."

Mary was relieved when other kidney function tests came back normal. After an evaluation, her doctors said she had a condition called, "proteinuria," the primary symptom of which is protein leaking out of the kidneys.

"They explained it to me using this metaphor: it's like you're making coffee and coffee grounds fall through the filter," she wrote. "I had faulty filters and they told me the situation wasn't that bad. But, while reassuring, doctors were using jargon and medical terms I'd never heard, and they were using it to describe me! It was disturbing. At the same time, I kept getting bigger and bigger, with water weight storing up inside me. I could hardly eat because there was no room in my abdomen for food. It was filled with fluid all around. It wasn't calories making me 'fat,' it was water. I was limited to only four glasses of fluid a day, but since it had nowhere to go, it was adding two pounds a day to my body. I gained 15 pounds in one week."

I interrupt Mary's narrative to share some scientific background of the disease that doctors believed she had. They read the results of a renal biopsy and diagnosed her with Minimal Change Disease (MCD). As its name implies, it isn't considered life-altering or life-threatening. When her kidney tissue was examined under a powerful microscope to observe a detailed anatomy of the glomeruli (again, the 'ball of yarn' in the kidneys), everything appeared normal. Studied under an electron microscope, which provided even greater magnification, the only abnormality was loss of space between the thin epithelial tissues on the border of the capillary loops.

The hardcore scientific explanation of MCD is that it's a condition characterized by effacement of the epithelial cell (podocyte) foot processes and loss of the normal charge barrier, such that albumin (a type of protein) selectively leaks out and proteinuria ensues. These "foot processes" do not refer to anything like the human foot, but to the base of these cellular structures. Protein sneaks through these structures when they're damaged.

Although usually seen in children, MCD can occur in adults. It initially presents with fluid retention, and often causes (as Mary experienced) swollen ankles and feet. The protein loss, coupled with increased blood levels of cholesterol defines nephrotic syndrome—Mary's initial diagnosis.

After nearly two years of being treated for MCD, however, her story darkened.

"During those two years, my doctors told me many times they were relieved that I 'only' had MCD," Mary wrote. "They said MCD was the most benign of kidney diseases, does not cause kidney failure, and often responds well to treatment. I heard repeatedly that I was lucky it wasn't something called FSGS, which I later learned stands for Focal Segmental Glomerular Sclerosis. Unfortunately, I was about to learn first-hand what FSGS can do to the human body."

During those first 24 months, when doctors still believed Mary only suffered from MCD, they administered a typical treatment of corticosteroids, even though the effectiveness of corticosteroids varies and often has substantive side-effects. Some patients show an immediate response—protein loss ceases and cholesterol levels normalize. Others become steroid sensitive, and though protein loss is reduced, even abated completely, it returns when steroids are discontinued. Very rarely, a patient is steroid-resistant and does not respond at all or only minimally to even high doses.

Mary's doctor started her on high-dose prednisone, but she continued spilling copious amounts of protein, which caused more fluid retention and severe bloating. Over time, prednisone changed the distribution of fat in her body—a new horror for Mary, as her body ballooned the same way her ankles had. She experienced a living nightmare, as water-filled fat-pads developed over her neck, and her entire body filled out like characters in the animated film, Shrek.

"In fact, around my daughter's friends I tried to make light of my new, huge body," she recalled. "They would just stare at me. I said I was trying out for the part of Fiona in a new Shrek movie. It made them laugh and relax, but inside I felt devastated.

"Over a period of three months, I gained fifty pounds of fluid that bulged from every inch of my body. My skin was stretched so tight I couldn't bend my legs to walk or get in or out of my car. My eye sockets protruded. My eyes were slits. I could barely see. So much fluid filled my body cavity I could hardly breathe. I looked nine months pregnant, but this wouldn't end with a bundle of joy. When I lay down at night, fluid leaked from my eyes because it had nowhere else to go. I despaired and felt it would never end. Doctors feared I might drown if the fluid leaked into my lungs."

Unfortunately, Mary's relationship and communication with her doctors were not at levels we promote in this book, making her situation much more difficult.

"Clearly, any patient going through what I was going through will have serious psychological and emotional challenges," Mary wrote. "And, none of the medical staff particularly cared about that. No one ever asked me how I was feeling emotionally, as if it didn't matter. Well, it did matter, it mattered a great deal. As a woman, it was especially difficult. While most of my friends were dieting and obsessed with calories, I gained 50 pounds almost overnight. This wasn't about vanity, it was about emotional survival. In public, I didn't want people to look at me. I felt humiliated, disoriented.

"I tried to continue with my life and my work, but I was so huge I couldn't sit comfortably to see clients. Moreover, they'd have been totally distracted by my distorted features and palpable suffering. I'm sure they would have wondered how I could counsel them when I obviously had my own issues. I still had to be mom and take my daughter to school functions, but even there, people would look away as if horrified by what they saw. I imagined they must be thinking I was sitting on the couch all day eating Bonbons. No matter how much I talked to myself and tried to maintain a positive attitude, I felt ashamed by the way I looked. I needed help to deal with this, and received none, zero, zip, from the medical staff. They didn't see me as a suffering person. They saw me as a kidney that was working abnormally."

Frustration, debilitation, and anguish dominated Mary's next two years, as powerful immunosuppressant drug treatments rendered no positive, or even encouraging, results. In fact, at this stage in her illness, the numerous drugs she was on created more ill effects than the disease itself. Making matters worse, they were all completely ineffective. Her physicians grew frustrated and concerned as well, as "textbook" MCD cases suggested she should, by now, have responded.

Mary's misery aside, it was starting to make them nervous.

Mary's mood swung from somewhat hopeful before a treatment to despair after failure to respond. Steroids, of course, can cause violent mood shifts and depression themselves, so Mary was bombarded on all sides. She felt weak, sluggish, depressed, and frightened. It wasn't until months later that an internist happened to mention to her that she could have her weight greatly reduced through a procedure at the hospital that would give her temporary relief until the pounds of fluid accumulated again.

"All this time I suffered great misery and embarrassment due to my weight gain and they could have done something about it, if only one of my doctors had mentioned it to me," she wrote. "It's hard to forget something like that. You try not to be resentful because it doesn't do you any good, but it's also hard to forget they let me suffer needlessly. I've learned you must take stands for what you need when you are on the 'medical conveyor belt,' because doctors don't always think holistically. They often only think of you like a mechanic thinks about a car, just a sum of mechanical parts."

In November 2008, Mary developed an upper respiratory infection, treated with antibiotics. Two weeks later, for the first time, her serum creatinine rose to 1.8 from her baseline of 1.2. Her urine now contained red blood cells and white blood cells. For the third, nerve-racking time, Mary traveled to Cedars Sinai Medical Center in Los Angeles for a renal biopsy. This time, the results came back with heart-wrenching results. Indeed, she had Focal Segmental Glomerulosclerosis (FSG), a disease that can initially mimics MCD, the disease she was told she was lucky she didn't have.

"That diagnosis put me on the highway to hell," she wrote. "They still had no idea what caused my kidney disease in the first place and now, after two years, they were telling me I had been misdiagnosed and had something worse.

"Despite the incredibly depressing new diagnosis, one wonderful thing happened to me, at this point," Mary said. "I met a doctor in the hospital doing weekend rounds, covering patients for the other doctors in town. I remember he sat down, took the time to talk to me, and then gave me a hug. To this day, the memory makes me emotional. Finally, somebody understood how much I was suffering, and actually cared. That's right, it was Dr. Fisher. He was my fourth doctor, but I knew immediately he was the one I needed."

Mary was so upset when I first saw her in the hospital, I knew something had to be done. Doctors don't equate emotional health with physical health often enough, but it has always been a part of my practice. It was easy to tell that Mary couldn't adequately fight her physical challenges until she was able to find trust and peace with her doctors. She was sensitive and intelligent, and I could literally see tension ease out of her body when she found someone listening to her.

She explained her frustrations and I listened until she was finished. Then I slowly began to share with her that if a renal biopsy doesn't penetrate deeply enough to obtain tissue from "juxta-medullary glomeruli" located deep in the kidney, FSG may not be seen, resulting in misdiagnosis of MCD. I could tell Mary appreciated the fact that I respected and cared about her as a person, but she was not at all impressed with my explanation. She remained angry that she had been misdiagnosed for so long, particularly given the ill-effects of all the medications she'd been given. Who could blame her?

I saw Mary occasionally on hospital rounds and eventually I became her nephrologist. She did everything we asked of her, but her nephrotic syndrome continued to worsen. It wasn't long before I knew we had to change our treatment course. I had to act. Mary had grown diuretic-resistant, so I initiated transient dialysis to remove large amounts of fluid and make her more comfortable. Her mood visibly brightened after that, as her figure slimmed down.

Cedars Sinai had experienced some success treating FSG with a protocol of plasmapheresis, plus infusions of intravenous immunoglobulin (IVIG) and a monoclonal antibody called Rituximab. Mary had several treatments utilizing this regimen, which left her drained and wrung out, limp as a rag doll. After a few weeks it became apparent this wasn't working.

"Nothing was easy during this time of misdiagnosis and treatments that didn't work," wrote Mary. "It was frustrating and frightening because none of these doctors could figure out what exactly was wrong and what to do about it. Dr. Fisher remained in my corner through it all. My husband was very generous with his time and efforts. He took me back and forth to the hospital, a two-hour drive each way. But, I could tell this was wearing him out emotionally. It was wearing me out, too."

Then, during one visit, doctors told her that her kidneys had failed completely.

"I was numb," she wrote. "They told me I had to start dialysis if I wanted to live. But, I didn't want to live. Not like that. What saved me was motherhood. My daughter needed me in her life. I had to live. But, it was very difficult. I felt terrible."

At first, Mary chose peritoneal dialysis, so she wouldn't have to depend on a dialysis center for treatment. Radiologists inserted a peritoneal catheter in her lower abdomen and she came home the same day. Ten days later, she used the catheter at the Santa Barbara Artificial Kidney Center, during the first of several training sessions. She told me later that, for her, peritoneal dialysis was a mistake. By doing it herself, she had effectively turned her house into a hospital room full of equipment.

Peritoneal dialysis required her to connect a tube that exited her abdomen from her peritoneal cavity. She learned to hook up to her peritoneal cycling machine every night. With time, her weight dropped and her energy rose along with her red-blood-cell count. She received intravenous iron and erythropoietin injections to further normalize her blood count (and hemoglobin level) so she could recoup some vitality. With a year of Vitamin D replacement to boot, she attained metabolic balance.

Dialysis is such a dramatic, life-saving process, such a leap forward in medical history, its genesis deserves a short discussion here. Consider, for example, the dialysis machine's inventor, because few people know about him, even though his story is as unlikely as it is remarkable. Dutch physician, Dr. Willem Kolff built the first dialysis machine during WWII. By all accounts, he was not only a technical genius, he exhibited extraordinary compassion for his patients, a compassion that drove his relentless work during and after the war. After building that first, crude dialysis machine (its initial parts, scavenged from junk yards, included sausage skin and orange-juice cans), he buried it in pieces around Holland, to keep occupying Nazi forces from discovering his invention. When the war ended, he dug up the parts, put them together and began using the resulting machine to sustain life. His first patient, ironically, was an elderly Nazi woman. Today, his vision has been refined into what Mary and millions of others use to stay alive.

With her enormous fluid overload reduced, Mary's life seemed a bit brighter. Still, she detested dialysis. Our discussions turned to transplantation. Even though patients with FSG risk a 30% chance of its recurrence in a transplant, Mary didn't look at it that way. To her, it meant she had a 70% chance to succeed. It was typical of her and many of patients to think that way. After years of misery, discouragement, and failed treatments, taking the risk was a no-brainer, and Mary took all the right steps to get on the waiting list for a new kidney.

"This gave me new hope, but I still needed to get through each day," she recalled. "One thing I learned to do, and this was critical to keeping myself together emotionally, was to stay focused on the present. I couldn't think too much about the future, dwell on the past, or fall into self-pity about why this was happening to me. That's a path to nowhere. I made dialysis and the other medical procedures part of my everyday routine, and tried to live life as normally as possible."

Then it happened. Meghan, a warmhearted friend of Mary's, volunteered to donate a kidney. A moment of exhilaration ensued as Mary awaited results of compatibility tests. Sadly, this feeling quickly faded when results showed that she and her friend were immunologically incompatible, a gap that would cause Mary's body to reject Megan's kidney.

Mary's heart sank, but doctors explained that there was still cause for hope. Mary and Meghan were allowed to participate in UCLA's Donor Exchange/Transplantation Program, which makes transplantation possible for incompatible donors by exchanging with another pair to transplant the most biologically compatible kidney into each recipient. Though recipients don't directly receive kidneys from their original, intended donors, all parties get what they want—donors donate and 'their' recipients receive the gift of life. This "paired exchange" technique is a beautiful mathematical algorithm that's changed the dynamics of kidney transplantation, lending renewed, realistic hope to patients worldwide.

Finally, the sun shone on Mary. A compatible donor in Fresno, California agreed to give her kidney to Mary, while Meghan's kidney would go to a patient with whom she was compatible. On October 23, 2010, Mary was admitted to UCLA Medical Center, where she received specialized infusions followed by a successful transplant.

"When I came out of the recovery room, the doctors were ecstatic," Mary recalled. "They were all telling me what a success it had been. One of them told me, 'Your kidneys work better than mine do.' I couldn't believe it. All that I had suffered seemed worthwhile now. I was going to live a normal life! I was thrilled beyond description.

"I was in a dream-like state for nearly 48 hours, finally allowing myself to picture a future where words like dialysis, protein leakage, and renal biopsies were relics of the past, I was euphoric until a doctor, with a grim look on his face, entered my room. 'The results of your last test just came back, and they are not good,' he said. 'Your FSG is back.' Thud. My heart crashed through the floor. I felt like the most cursed, wretched human on the planet. It was the darkest, grimmest, most dire day of my life. I was brought to my knees again, but this time I had no options. Doctors told me another transplant would likely have the same result, immediate return of FSG. They had no answers for me. They told me I had to 'be patient' and 'wait' until 'they' (whoever 'they' were) understood how to get this disease into remission. I had no faith in any of them or in my own future."

Mary's future turned into a bitter repetition of the past. She once again reluctantly accepted aggressive immunotherapy, making her feel like a blowfish, but after several treatments showed no improvement.

"When the new kidney finally failed, I wound up on dialysis again and I've been on it to this day," she writes. "On reading this, you'd think I am simply holding on, praying for the creation of an artificial kidney that might give me that part of my life back. But, things have changed for me, in a dramatic way. And maybe it's this change that made Dr. Fisher think my story is worth telling. Physically, of course, I would very much like things to change and to have a functioning kidney again. Yet, I am getting by. No one would mistake me for Fiona from Shrek anymore and I have taken on new challenges in my life, like writing a book and planning another one. But, here's the amazing part. I'm happier right now than I've ever been in my life! I'm more fulfilled and excited about life than I was before I knew I had a kidney problem. I want to explain to you, if I can, how this complete change came about. What I do know is that pain and despair can be great teachers, if you don't give into them. As Walt Disney once noted, you may not know it at the time, but a kick in the teeth may be the best things that ever happened to you.

"It began in the days and weeks following my failed transplant. The cold, hard, fact confronting me was that no one could help. Dr. Fisher was always there for me, but I realized the only thing that was going to make me 'better,' was within me—my relationship with life, my circumstances, and ultimately myself. I faced an inner spiritual challenge that would involve rising above my condition to find peace.

"It crystalized just when things were at their worst, when it seemed I had little to live for, other than my daughter. I was talked into taking a trip to Brazil. Brazil? I thought, when a friend asked me to go there with her. I'm battling a serious disease; how can I possibly think about trip like that? Yet, my own desperate circumstances ultimately motivated me to go. Why not? What's to lose?

"As some of you may know, there is a meeting place in Brazil for people from around the globe who are suffering, usually from a physical ailment not cured by traditional doctors. I met many wonderful people there and gave myself time to really think about life, what I was going through, and how I could change things to find happiness in my everyday existence, rather than stress and despair. Things changed then. I felt myself opening up to all circumstances in my life, accepting my kidney situation and then, taking a step further, I came to embrace life itself.

"Being brought to my knees in utter surrender, was, in large part, one of the best thing that has happened to me. It ignited the internal changes I made, which included not conjuring up ridiculous things to worry about. I took inventory of my strengths, courage, and capabilities. That was a positive step because it gave me a much stronger sense of self. I stopped spending time on everyday problems and hurdles. I just worked them out. No biggie. Cakewalk. I've got it. Other people's judgments of me didn't matter anymore, not after what I had been through and overcome. I gained the conviction that I have the right to live my life on my own terms. I learned to appreciate my body—how hard it has fought, and is fighting, to work while a machine keeps me going. Hating my body was a huge waste of energy, just because it didn't look the way I thought it should. Now, I'm grateful for how good it's been to me, which I acknowledge regularly.

"I've learned that gratitude is the key to a happy life. It's impossible to simultaneously feel grateful and badly. And, here's the best part of what I've learned: Gratitude is simple. It's a choice. I could feel bitter and despondent over being stuck on dialysis, or damn lucky because there is such a thing as dialysis. I could stew in envy that others have good health, or be happy that I'm doing as well as I am. I could lament that I can't accept an invitation to join my friends on their exotic sailing trips all over the world, or rejoice that I'm 'stuck' in a beautiful place that I call home. I now have this down to such an art, I find giddy appreciation in the simplest things, like being able to pee a little bit.

"Life doesn't go on forever. I now relish sweet moments with friends and family, the fresh smell of eucalyptus on my morning walk, the delicate breeze caressing and cooling my skin. 'This. Is. It', I think to myself. 'Drink it in, baby!' Dr. Fisher is still my kidney doctor. Finding a supportive doctor may be one of the most important things you do, as a patient."

Mary's metamorphosis from a fearful, angry, desperate, hopeless, person into an empowered one who has embraced life's opportunities, epitomizes the human spirit unleashed.

It's been ten years since the onset of her illness, but she has grown, emotionally and spiritually, beyond what most people achieve in their lifetimes. She has found courage and the will not just to live, but to feel grateful for what she has, to appreciate the little things, to love and be loved. Above all else, this is what I've so admired in my patients over the years.

"You don't need to suffer to deserve happiness," Mary concludes. "But, if you're suffering, just know that some of the most important lessons and joys of our lives can come out of that. Put aside despair and believe that you will arrive at a new place, one filled with sunlight, hope, and love, including love for yourself and your amazing body that fights so hard for you. Not easy, I know, but it's worth the struggle. The best feelings and understandings in life are waiting for you."

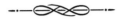

Chapter 6

Ed and Bill

My wife Leslie and I are confessed Volvo addicts, especially wagons, which we consider the safest family cars on the road. So, when we met with Bill Theurer at the Volvo dealership in Santa Barbara, we figured to bargain for another one.

We discussed the price of a car we liked and made an offer. Then came that awkward moment when Bill couriered that offer into the manager's office, for "Mr. Big's" review. A few minutes later, Bill came out smiling.

We had a deal.

Thus began a relationship that would uncannily draw Bill from the Volvo sales lot to my office, and draw us into a profound liaison, jump-started by a simple car deal and a strong handshake.

Meanwhile, Dr. Tom Allyn had recently arrived from Boston, where he served as chief of nephrology at Mount Auburn Hospital, to join my Santa Barbara practice. We enjoyed discussing mutual patients, exchanging ideas and creating a system for continuity of care. Sharing information enabled us to cover for each other during vacations, ensuring we understood treatment courses for each other's patients.

One afternoon, Dr. Allyn and I reviewed the case of a young man who presented with kidney failure. Ed Theurer, Bill's brother, displayed abnormal renal function and had recently undergone a diagnostic kidney biopsy that confirmed **hereditary nephritis**. Ed's dad, it seems, died young from kidney disease in the 1950s, before dialysis, transplantation, or any effective treatment for ESRD. Ed's diagnosis, therefore, clearly pointed to family history.

Uremic and feeling crappy, Ed presented with everything you'd expect—GFR less than 10cc/min., no appetite, weak, sleep deprived, short of breath. Worse yet, he'd smoked heavily for years—a poor choice that would ultimately pile more challenges onto a challenging situation. But for now, he needed dialysis. Fast.

Like most dialysis patients, Ed felt somewhat better after a few treatments. His uremic "fog" lifted and his previously impaired cognition improved. Still, even when given simple educational material like, "When Your Kidneys Fail" (published by the National Kidney Foundation), he lacked the attention span to understand it. Explanations of what had just happened to him and how he'd have to adopt a rigorous new lifestyle drifted hazy and lifeless through the air, like so much cigarette smoke. A nutritionist, critical to patient education about fluid restriction and reducing potassium and phosphorous intake, made no headway, either.

(When we hear "nutritionist," we typically think of somebody associated with a gym or weight-loss center. But highly trained nutritionists in a dialysis center serve a role as important as doctors or nurses. Put bluntly, if patients don't heed their guidance, they can die.)

Complicating matters, Ed started dialysis 28 years ago, when advanced, modern equipment and advanced therapeutic medications didn't exist. Inefficient, imprecise dialysis machines couldn't deliver a smooth procedure. Remember Mick's description of dialysis in 1979? Well, like Mick, Ed suffered horrible cramps, the kind dialysis patients describe as the most painful experience they've ever endured.

While uneven fluid removal contributed to Ed's cramps (and sudden blood-pressure drops, or "crashes"), so did a lack of self-control. He just couldn't reduce his fluid intake, which meant removing more of it on dialysis. Sometimes Ed arrived for treatment ten pounds above his "dry weight." Removing that much extra weight in a single, three or four-hour treatment to reduce blood pressure and keep fluid out of the lungs severely punishes the body, especially when repeated every two or three days.

Swell up, squeeze out, swell up, squeeze out—not good.

Sticking with admittedly tough dietary and fluid guidelines, instead, proves far safer and ultimately more comfortable than drinking and eating whatever you like when your kidneys don't work. That's a recipe for disaster. Clearly, Ed needed to gain control. He needed to comply.

To comply or not comply, that is the question. It's also the nephrologist's mantra and a patient's imperative to drink less, avoid certain foods, and take all prescribed medicines. You know from Chapter Two, it's not easy. In fact, it's damned hard. The sheer number of problems associated with ESRD—physical, psychological, social, nutritional—can overwhelm both patient and family during early months of treatment, from hospitalization, to catheter placement, to dialysis.

Thanks to persistent doctors, nurses and nutritionists, most patients overcome their confusion, dismay, and anger and eventually comply— the first, indispensable step toward improved health and a possible kidney transplant.

These days, due to increasing demand for transplants and a paucity of available kidneys, transplant centers weigh heavily a patient's compliance when evaluating qualifications to be placed on the national transplant list. It's not discriminatory, just discretionary, since transplant success depends in large part on a patient's strict adherence to direction, compliance with medicine regimens and regular follow-ups with the physician team.

Ed felt better after starting treatments, but like so many patients, soon resented his new life. He felt dependent, almost helpless, tied to tubes, machines, and other people's directives— repugnant notions for a man who formerly charted his own trajectory. He couldn't work due to scheduling problems and feeling irrepressibly ill. Financial stress heaped on more anxiety.

Ed had discussed renal transplantation with Dr. Allyn, but now, so frustrated with his life, he grew eager to find a donor or be placed on the transplant waiting list.

Ed spoke with his brother Bill, in seemingly good health and still working as sales manager at Volvo. Without hesitation, Bill agreed to donate to his ailing sibling. He called my office for a routine work-up, including blood draw and urinalysis.

At a follow-up appointment to review results, Bill sat in my waiting room, confident he could help his brother, whose suffering bothered him deeply. My secretary directed him into my office where I waited, worrying about how to confront him with some very disturbing news.

Not only could Bill not donate to Ed, his own creatinine was elevated. He, too, had kidney disease. With their family history—a dad who died from kidney failure and a brother with hereditary nephritis—Ed's lab results didn't wholly surprise me. We'd all just hoped for better.

I told Bill, "You're a special and courageous person, offering a kidney to your brother. And even though you feel well enough now to donate, it seems you've inherited the same disease."

Shocked and numb, Bill stared at me and through me, as if trying to grasp some ghostly, life-altering apparition. He'd seen his brother suffer, and now, through frightened, glazed eyes, he imagined himself in a similar mess.

Bill's creatinine level was 2.0, double his baseline level, meaning his kidneys were limping along at 50% function. If it doubled again to 4.0, his renal function would slip to 25%, edging toward full uremia. Like his brother before him, he was in trouble—bitter news for a man who entered the "kidney arena" with hopes of saving someone else.

Now, he'd have to save himself.

I discussed remaining blood-test results and completed a traditional medical history. We then went into the exam room for a complete physical evaluation. Bill had elevated blood pressure, but the rest of the exam was normal. He got dressed and we returned to the office to talk more.

By now, Bill had processed the news and anxiously shot-gunned questions my way. "Will I need to go on dialysis like my brother? Why do I feel so normal with such bad kidney disease? What can I expect to happen over the next few months?"

The more he queried, the more fear escalated in his voice. I created a timeline of a likely clinical course, with the caveat that it was only an estimate based on my knowledge of the natural history and progression of his disease.

"Bill. your kidney function will slowly decline over time, but we can delay the process a little by controlling your blood pressure" I told him. "If you reduce dietary salt and we add some medicine, your blood pressure will not be a problem. Beyond that, we'll periodically review your blood work to gauge the rate of progression." Before he left, I reminded Bill that he'd likely be a very good transplant candidate and by time he needed a kidney, transplant technology would be more advanced as well.

I wrote a prescription for blood-pressure meds and told Bill, "You have so much information to digest, let's reconvene in two weeks to check your BP and answer any further questions. Meanwhile, call me anytime to discuss your case."

Bill had been married for ten years when he learned that his kidneys were failing. Sadly, Bill had an unfulfilling marriage that ended in divorce. Fortunately, Bill and his wife had no children—kids who would have endured the double-whammy of divorce trauma and a chance of inheriting his disease.

Bill would remarry in 1994, his bride fully aware that he had progressive renal failure that would soon require dialysis. I didn't realize it at the time, but Bill had slumped into a state of denial about his disease. I didn't see him again for two years.

Ed, meanwhile, continued to struggle on dialysis. He smoked heavily, grew chronically depressed, and couldn't meet diet and fluid restrictions. Our staff spent enormous time educating him, but since Ed wasn't keen on verbalizing feelings, he got angry when pressed about compliance issues.

A brief note on smoking, the number one cause of preventable death in the United States: Despite false, immoral claims by big-tobacco companies and their lobbyists, tobacco will, in fact, kill you. Chew it, dip it, smoke it—it will kill you. It will destroy your heart, arteries, and lungs. If you dip or chew, the cancer it causes will eat your entire head, starting with your lip, cheek or jaw.

Wonder how I really feel about this body-and-soul-sucking habit and the mega-corporations that push it? About the same as I feel about companies pushing sugary foods that poison our youth and fuel the fire of epidemic obesity, which, in turn, fuels an ongoing epidemic of ESRD.

Okay, then, let's share a moment of smoking humor, as oxymoronic as that seems. I have a friend who always told his son, now 21, that smoking will kill you. Even when the boy was only seven, they played a word game about smoking. Dad would say, "You smoke. . ." and the boy would reply, "You die."

One night, when my friend's wife had convened her monthly book club, the young boy overheard a woman say, "I lost my cat to cancer this week." He immediately popped his innocent blond head up from behind a couch and asked, "Did your cat smoke?"
"I might have gone a bit too far," recalls his dad, "but I doubt he'll ever use tobacco."

Fortunately for Ed, his wife Gaylene, a nurse who worked in cardiology, understood complicated medical issues and was totally devoted to him. She alone could reach him when others failed, and his ability to endure dialysis resulted, in large part, from their love and her unwavering support.

Ed "hung in," and ultimately received a successful cadaveric transplant in 1999. Relief washed over Ed and Gaylene like a warm shower on a cold day. His new kidney functioned immediately, and after a few days Ed was home in Santa Barbara. But cryptic challenges lay ahead.

Ed's transplant continued functioning well, but he kept smoking and, shall we say, enjoyed his couch. Plus, like all transplant patients, he required high-dose immunosuppressants to ward off rejection and keep the kidney working—a trade-off by which a patient is more likely to develop cancer, especially skin cancer and lymphomas. And though Ed was already taking a statin drug to reduce high cholesterol levels, longstanding high blood pressure coupled with high cholesterol, smoking, and inactivity put him at great risk for cardiovascular disease down the road.

In 2006, seven years after his transplant, Ed felt pain in the left side of his lower abdomen that required hospital admission, where doctors diagnosed acute diverticulitis, a digestive disease involving inflammation of pouches within the large-bowel wall. They administered broad-spectrum antibiotics, intravenous fluids, and a no-eating directive.

The pain continued, however, and Ed's white-blood-cell count rose, indicating a severe infection that created a potential medical emergency. Drugs that prevented Ed's immune system from rejecting his kidney weakened his ability to combat the infection. A dreaded scenario loomed, a balancing act that, if it didn't work, could cost him his kidney, his life, or both. The question was this: Should we reduce prednisone and cyclosporine doses to allow Ed's immune system to effectively fight this life-threatening infection, even if it resulted in kidney rejection? We opted to save his life and hope the kidney survived.

Further complicating matters, imaging of Ed's abdomen revealed that his infected diverticulum had ruptured. Emergency surgery removed a large piece of infected colon and because of this operation, the surgeon had to create a colostomy, bringing a portion of the large intestine through the abdominal wall to carry stool from Ed's body.

The good news: Removing the inflamed, infected bowel, along with continued antibiotic treatment, saved Ed's life and spared his kidney. The bad news: Ed would live with a colostomy bag, a situation freighted with psychological consequences.

Ed regained his strength and energy, but it took months. Gaylene helped with colostomy care, medication compliance and doctors' appointments—all while providing the loving support he needed.

Three years later, Ed's chest-pain episodes began. He'd had many risk factors for cardiac disease and now they'd rolled back to him like the proverbial bad penny. His cardiologist suspected angina (pain caused by a blockage in one or more coronary arteries). An angiogram confirmed that Ed had severe coronary artery disease, requiring placement of four stents in affected blood vessels. Thankfully, Ed has been angina-free ever since.

For a body ravaged by vascular disease from smoking, high cholesterol, high blood pressure, and ESRD, atherosclerosis in blood vessels marches on. Ed's cardiologist, for example, ultimately discovered an aneurysm (a ballooning or stretching of a blood-vessel wall that may rupture under the pressure of blood flow) in a large artery supplying blood to his leg, the iliac artery. Doctors treated it with blood-pressure control and monitoring to make sure it didn't expand to a point of potential rupture.

Somehow, with confidence in his medical team and support from a steadfast wife, Ed processed each new challenge, accepted the threat and fought on. Sadly, however, he continued smoking, even when told it would accelerate his vascular disease.

He enjoyed a couple of uneventful years until doctors discovered a type of skin cancer called squamous cell—a common side effect of immunosuppression. A dermatologist went to work, and over time removed many squamous lesions. (I ask my transplant patients to see a dermatologist twice a year for a thorough skin inspection; some go every two months.) Ed now added a new chore to his medical to-do list.

Stability reigned again until a visit to Dr. Allyn revealed an unexpected rise in Ed's creatinine, again indicating a potentially devastating medical problem. Subsequent tests showed steadily worsening kidney function. Finally, a renal biopsy indicated no rejection, but evidence that vascular disease and hypertension had accelerated Ed's recurring renal failure.

Ed's courage, resilience and will to live remained strong, despite facing imminent dialysis after years of freedom. He began dialysis treatments, but soon after developed pneumonia. A CT scan showed his pneumonia improving, but, incredibly, it also showed a mass in his lung. A biopsy indicated squamous cell carcinoma, much like the skin cancers to which he'd been prone.

There was no time for depression, only action. How Ed mustered the energy and spirit to tackle this new, life-threatening problem, considering the previous cascade of medical catastrophes, defies credulity.

After visiting an oncologist, Ed started radiation therapy. Today, his tumor is shrinking after fourteen courses of laser therapy. Plus, until recently, Ed stubbornly refused to taper immunosuppressives that were partially responsible for his skin and lung cancers, because he believed his kidney function might return. Finally, we've tapered these medications and he has accepted his new reality.

And he finally quit smoking.

Dr. Allyn and I lost touch with Bill and he skipped follow-ups from 1992 to 1994. He returned to see me shortly after his wedding, complaining of fatigue, shortness of breath, poor appetite, nausea, insomnia, and low libido. His complexion was sallow; he looked exhausted and frail—not surprising, since his creatinine and BUN were 12.4 and 134, respectively. His Hemoglobin was 8.8, consistent with severe ESRD-related anemia.

Miserable as he was, Bill remained in denial about his dire situation, at first refusing dialysis. "Bill, go home," I told him, "Think about it. I know this is scary, but you've seen how well your brother has done. He went through the same process, and now he has a functioning transplant (this was before Ed's transplant succumbed to vascular disease). I'll call you in the morning. You'll feel so much better the sooner we deal with this."

Finally, Bill entered Cottage Hospital for catheter placement and initial dialysis. I did what I could to ensure an uneventful first treatment, considering Bill was so fragile and fearful. (If introduction to dialysis proves traumatic, it can create fear and distrust for every subsequent intervention.) I was waiting in the hospital's dialysis unit when he arrived. I smiled and reassured him that he would soon feel better. He seemed relieved to see me.

The acute hemodialysis nursing staff at Cottage Hospital have worked together for twenty-five years. They care for critically ill patients suffering from systemic problems that cause kidney failure, such as septic shock, heart failure, or bleeding from serious surgery. Their labor-intensive, stressful work requires considerable medical knowledge and experience. In addition, they see new patients recently diagnosed with chronic renal failure, delivering their first few dialysis treatments in a safe hospital setting before releasing them to outpatient care. That makes them experts, too, in managing patients' confusion and fear.

Dr. Allyn and I have served as Co-Medical Directors of Acute Dialysis at Cottage Hospital since 1982. We work seamlessly with a highly trained, expert, and empathetic nursing staff, resulting in minimal turnover and, importantly, efficient teamwork. Patients needing perfect continuity of care and crisp communication with health-care providers depend on it.

On admission, Bill had a litany of lab tests, including screening for hepatitis and HIV, which could infect a staff member who routinely encounters blood, plus coagulation studies to rule out bleeding disorders (uremic patients already display poorly functioning platelets, which may correlate with a propensity for bleeding).

Following placement of Bill's "perm-cath," he had his first hemodialysis treatment. The mantra for initial treatments is "slow is pro," as correcting metabolic abnormalities accumulated over years takes time. We treated Bill daily for short periods, gradually removing fluid with each treatment until his blood pressure began to normalize. Same with his metabolic abnormalities. We treated them little by little each day.

Home from the hospital, though feeling much better, Bill slammed headlong into emotional grief. His bride of only several months told him, "This is all too depressing for me," and left him. The sting of multiple losses, right when he was trying to recover and reorient his thinking and his life, left Bill as lonely as lonely gets.

Some dialysis patients, not all, literally fail to thrive. Bill continuously flirted with membership in this category. Lacking support of family and friends, a non-thriver may develop complicated medical issues and require more time and attention to help fill their emotional glass to "half-full."

Over the next four years, while caring for Bill's serious medical issues, I also felt like his motivator-in-chief. I tried to buoy his spirits and to make him believe he had some control over his destiny. I knew Bill would likely receive a kidney transplant if he could comply—stay in metabolic balance by drinking less fluid, taking dozens of necessary pills, and avoiding dangerous foods, especially potassium-rich foods. I preached patience and self-discipline to escape a situation he found vile.

Nephrologists' (and nurses') mentoring skills ultimately rank close to their medical skills, especially since kidney patients all experience negativity, anxiety, even depression at some point in their treatment. Patients in a prolonged negative mode are usually less compliant, too, and wind up in the hospital more frequently for acute problems like fluid in their lungs or life-threatening potassium levels.

Ways to address the stress of caring for fragile, complicated patients include monthly staff meetings. Nephrologist, nurse, physician assistant, dietician and social worker participate in these meetings, in which all patients' cases are reviewed. Everybody vents, without judgment, their frustration with non-compliant patients. This relieves stress, guides our treatment plans, and gets us all on the same "therapeutic page."

Bill had his brother and sister-in-law Gaylene for emotional support. Ed, with his excellent kidney transplant (at the time), demonstrated what was possible if Bill could be patient and disciplined. Still, it took a monumental team effort to keep Bill in stable health long enough to receive a kidney transplant.

Stuck in darkness, he struggled to see the light.

To liberate Bill from the dialysis center, he accepted a trial of peritoneal dialysis. His job was to complete at least four exchanges every day. He also needed to visit his physician at least once a month and frequently check with a PD nurse.

Bill had a PD catheter placed and was discharged the next morning. A week later, he began a training program and two weeks after that began PD at home—liberated from hemodialysis, but directed to follow strict, sterile protocols for this form of therapy.

At first Bill was elated because PD met his expectations. It was technically easy to do at home on Bill's schedule and allowed him to drink more fluid and eat some foods prohibited on hemodialysis. Life was getting better until Bill ran into the number one problem for PD patients: Recurrent infections resulting in peritonitis, an inflammation of the peritoneum, a thin tissue lining that covers the inside of the abdominal cavity.

One month into his treatments Bill called with abdominal pain. I asked him about the nature of fluid draining into his bag. He said it was cloudy—the first sign of what would be relentless staph aureus bacterial infections. A severe infection, peritonitis usually results from contamination of the peritoneal dialysis system. A skin organism like staphylococcus aureus enters the system in a variety of ways. Caught early and treated vigorously, it can usually be cured.

But not for Bill. For unexplained reasons, after using every "cure" in our medical bag, Bill's infection recurred with increasing frequency, causing pain, more hospitalizations, and more antibiotic treatments. He also exhibited very early scarring of his native peritoneal membrane, ultimately precluding him from continuing PD.

Quite discouraged, Bill grew negative and depressed again, like he'd been on hemodialysis. Worse yet, he lost massive amounts of protein that exited his inflamed peritoneal membrane during bouts of infection, leaving him weak as a kitten.

Bill headed back to hemodialysis, back to square one.

From 1994 through 1998, Bill fought hard to survive. Even though I was a good cheerleader, telling him it would not be much longer before he'd get an available kidney, he seemed to lose hope, and his lab results showed it. Bill was gaining more weight between treatments, forcing nurses to prolong the treatments and "pull" more fluid off each time. He felt more "washed out" after each treatment and grew more withdrawn.

On December 15, 1998, he arrived at hemodialysis and before we could get him started, he passed out. His blood pressure and heart rate were very low. Staff initiated CPR and drew blood. Paramedics rushed him to Cottage Hospital. On arrival, his blood pressure was unobtainable and his EKG revealed a developing sine wave, a finding reflecting a dangerously elevated serum potassium level (it was 8.2; normal is 3.6 to 4.8). Bill was intubated and placed on a breathing machine. The ER doctor and I lowered his potassium with drugs.

Bill's EKG improved as his potassium level fell. We began dialysis, which effectively removed the excess potassium from his blood, resulting in a normal cardiogram by the end of the treatment. He woke up and indicated that we should remove the breathing tube. The tube removed, he seemed alert and pain-free. He did not suffer any neurological damage. His recovery from near-death without harm to his heart or brain was the first good luck Bill had experienced in a long time.

He was alive, but now what?

Clearly, we'd failed to motivate him to "comply." He had indulged in high potassium foods that almost killed him. I practically pleaded with him to just be a little more patient. I recounted the story of a patient who had experienced similar difficulties and soon after received a new kidney and was thriving. Bill went home on this positive note.

I saw Bill in the dialysis a week later. He was a little better but still in shock from his cardiac ordeal. He planned a quiet weekend at home to celebrate Christmas. His phone rang at 3:00 am on Christmas morning. Bill opened his groggy eyes and answered. The voice on the other end said, "Bill, this is the transplant coordinator at Cedars Sinai Medical Center. We have a kidney for you and in fact it appears to be a perfect match. It is from a fourteen-year-old, who died of a gunshot wound to the head. Are you interested?"

Merry Christmas, indeed.

Bill arrived at Cedars at 6:00 am. His final hurdle was a cross-match test to ensure compatibility with the donor. It indicated that Bill did not form dangerous antibodies against the donor's blood and the transplant went forward. At the end of the procedure the new kidney began making clear, golden urine. Within four days, Bill enjoyed normal kidney function.

Twenty-five years later, Bill still enjoys perfect kidney function and an active life. He works and maintains a close relationship with his brother. And now he's the cheerleader, visiting a dialysis unit in Los Angeles, where he lives, encouraging patients with his story and the message that with hope, patience, and endurance, anything is possible.

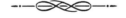

Chapter 7

Clare

Bounding by Jeep through the African savanna, Clare grabbed the vehicle's roll bar, stood up and looked around. To her left, elephants grazed in red-oats grass, occasionally flapping their giant ears to shed swarms of flies. To her right, giraffes stretched high to nibble leaves from the roofed dome of a baobab tree.

Protected from a flaring African sun by her neck-flap hat, Clare blinked twice, once to clear dust from her eyes, once to make sure she wasn't dreaming. The tear that beaded high on her cheek, in fact, could have been from either—the dusty, hot African day or completion of a life's journey that began several years prior in Santa Barbara.

Back then, Clare enjoyed work as a financial executive, raising two beautiful daughters, arcing from the mountains to the sea for exercise and adventure. Only one disaster occluded her sunny life: divorce, complete with lawyers and ugly settlement negotiations that tightened her gut and drained her so completely she could barely recall the day she said, "I do."

I asked Clare about stress before, during, and after the divorce. "I was fine until the whole ordeal," she said. "It was excruciatingly painful and debilitating, made worse by increasing stress at work. For months on end, I woke up every day to a mountain of anxiety."

A couple years of after she and her daughters soldiered through the crippling divorce, Clare awoke one day feeling tired and chilled. She dismissed these symptoms and went to work as usual. A viral infection, she figured, which would run its course. She worked through her fatigue over the next few days, but soon her muscles and joints felt achy and painful, symptoms prompting a visit to an internist. By then, she'd also developed a dry cough.

Clare's physical exam revealed no obvious problem, so she was advised to rest and told that most likely this "viral infection" would get better on its own. Instead, she got worse. Her body ached, her cough progressed, and eventually her doctor ordered blood tests that showed abnormal kidney function: slightly elevated creatinine with some protein and red blood cells in her urine.

That's when I first saw Clare. Like many patients referred to nephrologists, she had no idea she suffered from a virulent illness that could cause organ failure. Reviewing her medical history and blood-test results, her malady appeared to be glomerulonephritis, a nonspecific term describing inflamed glomeruli. Her cough, however, had grown more frequent, producing sputum. She'd also developed shortness of breath when active.

I sent her for a chest x-ray and more blood tests. The x-ray revealed opacities in both upper lung fields. Alarmingly, her creatinine had doubled; she'd rapidly lost 50% of her kidney function.

Whatever ailed Clare, it was coming on fast.

(Though physicians are taught to react dispassionately, intellectually, to a patient's developing clinical profile, gathering supportive evidence for diagnosis and treatment, I've always struggled to suppress my gut reaction to what I know will be arduous, dangerous, life-changing events. At times, this has tormented me. Other times, it's helped me bond with patients to elevate their hope and determination, partnering to advocate for and achieve successful outcomes. Often, it's done both.)

First, I needed to tell Clare what the data meant and how we could accurately diagnose her problem, which meant starting with a kidney biopsy. Delivering this information, possibly the first step in a long ordeal, takes delicacy, time, and considerable thought, balancing hope with logic, truth, and candor about dangers that procedures like this, or its results, might pose. I also needed to allay her manifest anxiety and get her to trust my judgment.

We had a long talk. I explained my conclusions, based on lab tests and symptoms. I tried not to overly alarm her, but she needed to understand that she had a serious illness affecting her kidneys and lungs, which required immediate diagnosis. I told her about a class of diseases that simultaneously affect both organs. It's called "Pulmonary-Renal Syndrome," usually caused by inflammation in small or medium-sized blood vessels in both organs.

The inflammation's cause remains unknown. We do know this, however: Without immediate treatment, the disease can progress rapidly and lead to kidney and lung failure.

I answered Clare's questions, relaying past experiences with patients who faced similar pulmonary/kidney issues. She absorbed the information, and by the nature of her questions I felt satisfied that she reasonably understood the challenges at hand.

The gnawing thought of a renal biopsy, having a needle inserted three times through her back muscles into the lower pole of a kidney to gather enough tissue for an accurate diagnosis, frightened Clare. As I've described, the procedure is generally safe, posing slight but real risks, especially excessive bleeding. Explaining this to a patient (a legal requirement in our increasingly litigious society) doesn't help calm them.

The biopsy was uneventful, with sufficient tissue removed for diagnosis. Clare went back to her room, where nurses monitored her for bleeding, but she complained of increasing shortness of breath. Were hyperventilation and anxiety causing this? Something worse?

It was worse. A nurse placed a pulse oximeter on the end of a finger to measure the amount of oxygen in her blood, which proved abnormally low. She needed oxygen, plus her blood pressure was climbing and her urine output diminishing. Clare was in serious trouble.

I ordered more blood tests, which indicated her kidney function had worsened. As Clare headed to Intensive Care, we sent tissue from her biopsy to Cedars Sinai, where world-class renal pathologist Dr. Arthur Cohen, would interpret the results.

But an ominous clock was ticking. To treat Clare before progressive disease permanently destroyed her kidneys, we needed information fast. So, besides sending the sample to Dr. Cohen, we prepared a slide of tissue from her biopsy for me to examine with our own pathologist. Though we don't perform elaborate stains necessary to make a specific diagnosis, we can immediately detect a rapidly progressive process.

I winced the moment I viewed a glomeruli-rich tissue sample. Sixty-six percent of 18 glomeruli were severely involved in a process manifested by angry-looking cells, literally marching from one end of the glomerulus to the other, filling the space normally meant for newly forming urine. This army of aggressive cells ravaged the units of function (glomeruli) responsible for the kidney's ability to cleanse blood. A couple days later, Dr. Cohen confirmed a diagnosis of "Rapidly Progressive Glomerulonephritis" that had already destroyed 90% of her glomeruli.

I knew Clare's chances of regaining kidney function were slim, but there was still a chance. When I explained the gravity of the problem to her, I don't think Clare fully understood it. She was young, previously healthy, and heard what she wanted to hear—that aggressive treatment might reverse the problem.

Clare received large intravenous doses of solumedrol, a potent steroid, for three straight days. Roughly equivalent to prednisone, milligram to milligram, one patient vividly remembers solumedrol. "It was in the old days," he recalls, "when right after a kidney transplant they infused you with 2,000 mg. of solumedrol. I'll never forget it. I sporadically awoke in ICU thinking I'd gone mad, literally insane. I was hallucinating like crazy, and alarms going off on other machines only aggravated my insanity. In my jangled, disoriented state, I remember thinking, 'What have I done; I never should have had this transplant.'"

Potent stuff, to say the least.

The rationale for Clare's treatment was this: if we could reduce the severe inflammation that was destroying her glomeruli, we could then give her Cytoxan, an immunosuppressant, that would attack the cause of the inflammation and arrest the process entirely.

During the first week of therapy, her lung function improved until she no longer needed oxygen. Sadly, her kidneys did not. I vividly remember the gravity and sullenness of our conversation when I explained to Clare that her disease was so virulent that our drugs couldn't restore kidney function. I didn't, however, rule out the possibility of some improvement. She held back tears, clinging, like fingernails on a mountainside, to inner strength and resolve.

Still, Clare was numb, drained from her recent travails. She absorbed the news silently, too perplexed to ask more questions. She hadn't had enough time to process what was happening to her. She got so sick so fast—uremic, gasping for oxygen, her body invaded by needles, a biopsy, and a large catheter placed in a vein beneath her collar bone for dialysis—how could she?

On the upside, her lungs were recovering. Dialysis would remove toxins from her body, improve her breathing, help improve her appetite and allow her body to rebuild strength after surviving a tempest.

When Clare arrived at the Santa Barbara Artificial Kidney Center, she was exhausted, depressed, and highly vulnerable to infection because she was still on high-dose steroids. Over time, we aimed to slowly taper these steroids, which kept her lung-function from worsening.

Clare had several daily dialysis treatments to remove excess fluid, reduce blood pressure and make breathing easier. Her mood remained flat, but she enjoyed great support from friends, especially from her daughters, who always lifted her spirits.

Then it happened, like it does for many dialysis patients who suffer through months or years of torment—a lightning bolt of grace, a cloudburst of good fortune. Clare's sister came forward to offer a kidney.

The transplant went seamlessly. The new kidney functioned immediately, donor and recipient emerging with no ill effects. Clare celebrated her newfound freedom. Transplants are unique this way. To feel so chronically sick, to flirt with death, then suddenly, boom, you're well again. With more than a hint of irony, transplant patients "describe" this feeling of restored health as "indescribable."

Equally devastating, however, is the fall when a transplant fails. This was Clare's fate. Soon after her transplant, a urinalysis revealed the dreaded appearance of protein. She had a viral infection that strongly correlates with transplant rejection. It's called parvovirus, not uncommon in severely immunosuppressed patients.

Antiviral medication was administered immediately. Nonetheless, Clare's kidney function slowly waned, along with her mood. When it was clear she was headed back to dialysis, we discussed the future. I told her we'd would work together to stabilize her health, get her off anti-rejection drugs, and get her well-nourished in preparation for another transplant.

I offered anecdotes of patients who'd endured rejections but thrived with another transplant. I've found this approach, this information, effective in equipping a grieving patient with hope, belting them in for the pilgrimage to a second kidney.

Clare started dialysis again, and in October 2003, doctors removed her transplanted kidney due to a persistent low-grade fever linked to ongoing rejection. Her fever abated, but she continued fighting infections like sinusitis, leaving her in a near-constant malaise.

Due to Clare's recurrent infections, I measured her blood-level of gamma globulin, a protein that fights off infections and supports the immune system. It was very low. On dialysis, she then received monthly intravenous gamma globulin replacement, keeping her infection-free.

Clare resolved to eat well, exercise, and do all she could to remain healthy and ready for another kidney. She'd seen the Holy Land and was dead-set on returning there. Her self-discipline was royally rewarded when a friend came forward to give Clare a new kidney and another shot at a normal life.

In 2005, Cedars Sinai was at the cutting edge of transplant technology, starting induction therapy with intravenous gamma globulin, rituximab, and plasmapheresis to remove unwanted antibodies that might cause transplant rejection. Remember Mick? Well, like Mick, Clare had been "sensitized" from her previous transplant, dangerous antibodies lurking in her blood, ready to attack a new kidney.

Clare received the pre-transplant therapy, and on August 3, 2005, she received her friend's kidney, enjoying normal function within a few days. She felt ineffable gratitude for her heroic friend but she knew, most certainly, that the future is uncertain.

Thankfully, though, life went on as if she'd never been sick. Clare met her daughter's future husband and helped plan their wedding, an especially joyful event for a family that had seen little joy for so long. Grandchildren that followed inspired and energized Clare, who now spends many pleasure-filled hours with them.

There was, however, a period, common among transplant recipients, when anxiety, centered around the fear of losing her kidney, plagued her. With time, however, anxiety abated, replaced by everyday vigilance and awareness of her physical state.

That vigilance paid off some months later, when Clare told me she'd been coughing. A chest x-ray revealed a round lesion called a nodule in her right upper lung field. Among immuno-suppressed patients like Clare, unusual infections can always occur, as can cancer.

Fear and anxiety returned.

Clare, it turns out, had developed a Cryptococcus infection, a fungal disease we effectively treated with antibiotics for eight months. Her kidney remained safe, the disease has not recurred, and the merry-go-round of fear, anxiety, wellness, and confidence circled back to the happier side of life.

Eight years later, Clare's kidney still functions perfectly. She recently returned from her African safari, about as far from illness and the life-sustaining necessities of dialysis as you can get.

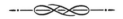

Chapter 8

Henry

Henry understood clearly the road connecting obesity, diabetes, dialysis, and death. He'd already lost two older brothers to complications from the disease, each enduring ESRD, then fatal heart attacks.

Henry, also diabetic, started down a similar path, suffering ESRD in 1998. Like his brothers, he loved eating foods dense in sugar and calories, but void of much nutritional value. Consequently, he too was quite overweight.

Would he join his siblings on that tragic highway?

After a short time on dialysis, Henry received a deceased-donor kidney in 1999. His creatinine settled in at 1.3, near-perfect function. Gratefully unchained from dialysis, he wanted to help children in the Latino community avoid the medical problems that killed his brothers and stole his kidney function.

When I started the Diabetes Resource Center (DRC), I thought that if community members like Henry, who became obese and developed diabetes, could educate with their stories, they might effectively help families reverse poor lifestyle habits and the path to this debilitating disease.

Henry stepped up, and into the role of "Promotoro de Salud." He helped many children learn to eat better and understand potential consequences of obesity. When local TV anchor Debby Davison did a story about the importance of preventing childhood obesity and its role in causing diabetes, she focused on the DRC. To Henry's delight, she interviewed him.

But type 2 diabetes never disappears. It slowly and methodically injures small blood vessels that nurture all organ systems. Despite the benefits of a kidney transplant, Henry evidenced all the typical complications. Diabetes affected his vision, requiring many laser treatments to prevent blindness. Before his kidneys failed, he suffered severe angina (chest pain) caused by blocked coronary arteries. He even had a five-vessel coronary bypass a couple of years before starting dialysis.

Due to a family history of diabetes that irrevocably ended in early death, Henry didn't think he'd live too long, despite his excellent new kidney. My job was to empower him to keep his blood-sugar levels as close to normal as possible, maintain perfect blood pressure, and continue to control his cholesterol levels in a desired range.

In 2010, eleven years after his transplant, Henry's creatinine remained at 1.3 with no new cardiac issues. He did his best to maintain his blood sugar in the target range—a considerable challenge, to say the least. Then, for the first time, a trace of protein showed up in his urine. This either meant rejection, or that diabetes was damaging his kidney. A renal biopsy suggested the latter. We undertook a huge effort to gain better control of Henry's blood sugar. He'd been insulin-dependent and now required more, despite a respectable diet.

Henry and his kidney hung in there, but in September 2011, short of breath, Henry suffered heart failure. A test called a thallium scan that images the heart after injection of adenosine, a drug used to help assess cardiac function, suggested that he had severe, inoperable small-vessel disease.

For the next four years, we struggled with many consequences of Henry's severe diabetes, which attacked blood vessels in his heart and lower extremities. It also caused his heart muscle to slowly degenerate, making it unable to adequately pump blood to his kidney and other organs. For example, he developed gangrene of the right foot, which required amputation of his toes.

During this time, however, his iron-willed kidney never fully failed.

In 2015, Henry developed pain in his left foot and leg. He underwent successful "revascularization" to improve blood supply to his left lower extremity. A week later, however, he came to the ER with pain and redness in his leg. His blood pressure dropped suddenly and doctors couldn't resuscitate him. His kidney was still functioning when he died.

Henry lived to 78, far exceeding his brothers' lifespans. He enjoyed many very good years with family, thanks to his kidney transplant and the modicum level of metabolic balance it afforded. Still, his story underscores diabetes' devastating effects and reminds that this pernicious disease is growing to epidemic proportions in the 21st century.

Reducing the incidence of diabetes should be a top national and personal health-care priority. Otherwise, like it's physiological partner obesity, our health-care system and health-care budget may bloat beyond repair.

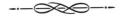

Capítulo 8

Henry

Henry entendió claramente el camino que conecta la obesidad, diabetes, diálisis y la muerte. Ya había perdido a dos hermanos mayores de complicaciones de la enfermedad, cada uno de insuficiencia renal causando ataques al corazón fatales. Henry, también diabético, iniciado por un camino similar, padeciendo de fallo renal en 1998. Como sus hermanos, le encantaba comer alimentos densos en azúcar y calorías, evitando comidas mas nutritivas. A consecuencia, termino el también con bastante sobrepeso. ¿¿ terminaría el por el mismo camino como sus hermanos? Después de un corto tiempo en diálisis, Henry recibió un trasplante de riñón cadavérico en 1999. Su creatinina se estanco en 1.3, lo cual indicaba que tenia función casi perfecta. Agradecido inmensamente y completamente desatado de diálisis, se propuso a ayudar a los niños en la comunidad Latina a evitar los problemas médicos que mataron a sus hermanos y le robó su función renal. Cuando empecé la el centro de diabetes, pensé si podríamos educar a los miembros de la comunidad como Henry, con sus historias, su experiencia podrían efectivamente ayudar a las familias revertir hábitos de vida pobres y el camino a esta debilitadora enfermedad...

Henry, se animo y empezó el papel de "Promotor de Salud." Él ayudó a muchos niños a aprender a comer mejor y a comprender las posibles consecuencias de la obesidad. Cuando una presentadora de TV local hizo una historia sobre la importancia de prevenir la obesidad infantil y su papel en la causa de diabetes, se enfoco en nuestro centro de diabetes. Para deleite de Henry, ella lo entrevistó.

Pero la diabetes tipo 2 nunca desaparece. Lentamente y metódicamente lesiona los vasos sanguíneos pequeños que nutren todos los sistemas de los órganos. A pesar de las ventajas de su trasplante de riñón, Henry fue desarrollando todas las complicaciones típicas y comunes de la diabetes. Diabetes afecto su vista, necesitando muchos tratamientos de laser para prevenir la ceguera. Antes de que sus riñones fallaron, Henry sufrió (dolor del pecho) causada por el bloqueo de las arterias coronarias. Incluso tuvo un desvió coronario donde se bloquearon cinco vasos sanguíneos lo cual ocurrió un par de años antes de comenzar la diálisis.

Debido a antecedentes familiares de diabetes que irrevocablemente terminó en muerte temprana, Henry no creía que viviría mucho tiempo, a pesar de su nuevo riñón que trabajaba súper bien. Mi trabajo como medico consistía en inculcarle a él para mantener sus niveles de azúcar en la sangre lo mas normal posible, mantener una presión arterial ideal y mantener los niveles de colesterol en un rango deseado.

En 2010, once años después de su trasplante, creatinina de Henry se mantuvo en 1,3 y no tenía nuevos problemas cardiacos. Él hizo su mejor esfuerzo para mantener su azúcar en la sangre en el rango deseado, lo cual era un reto enorme, por decirlo asi. Entonces, por primera vez, un rastro de proteína se empezó a aparecer en su orina. Esto significó rechazo o diabetes estaban dañando su riñón.

Una biopsia renal sugirió que era la diabetes. Se realizó un gran esfuerzo para obtener mejor control de azúcar en la sangre de Henry. Había sido dependiente de insulina y ahora requería más y mas insulina, a pesar de llevar una dieta respetable.

Henry y su riñón se mantuvieron al margen, pero en Septiembre de 2011, con mucha falta de aliento, Henry entra en insuficiencia cardíaca. Un examen llamado un thallium scan que revela imagines del corazón después de la inyección de **adenosina**, un medicamento utilizado para ayudar a evaluar la función cardiaca, sugirió que tenía una enfermedad de los pequeños vasos sanguíneos, la cual era inoperable.

Para los próximos cuatro años, luchamos con muchas consecuencias de la diabetes, que atacaba los vasos sanguíneos en su corazón y las extremidades de los pies. También causó que su que músculo cardíaco se degenerara lentamente, lo que es incapaz de bombear adecuadamente la sangre a su riñón y otros órganos vitales. A consecuencia de esto, Henry desarrolló gangrena del pie derecho, que requirió la amputación de los dedos del pie.

Durante este tiempo, sin embargo, su riñón de hierro nunca le fallo.

En el año 2015, Henry desarrolló dolor en su pie izquierdo y la pierna. Se tuvo q someter una cirugía donde se revascularizo su circulación y esta fue todo un éxito para mejorar la circulación a la extremidad baja del lado izquierdo. Una semana más tarde, sin embargo, llegó a la sala de urgencias con dolor y enrojecimiento en la pierna. Su presión arterial cayó repentinamente y los médicos no pudieron reanimarlo. Su riñón estaba funcionando aún cuando murió.

Henry vivía a 78, lo que supera la vida de sus hermanos. Disfrutó de muchos años muy buena con la familia, gracias a su trasplante de riñón y el nivel mínimo de equilibrio metabólico que brinda. Sin embargo, su relato subraya que los efectos de la diabetes son devastadores y recuerda que esta enfermedad perniciosa crece a proporciones de epidemia en el siglo 21st .

La reducción de casos de diabetes debe de ser una prioridad superior personal y nacional. De lo contrario, tanto la obesidad que es un hermano fisiológico de la diabetes quebraran nuestro sistema de salud y presupuesto financiero al punto que no pueda ser reparado.

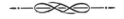

Chapter 9

Philip

Born in Minnesota, Philip attended Westmont College and has remained in the Santa Barbara area, working as a successful accountant. He enjoyed excellent health until 1997, when he experienced decreased hearing and a peculiar ringing in his left ear.

An MRI confirmed a tumor called an acoustic neuroma, generally benign and accessible to surgery. During Philip's preoperative physical exam, however, doctors felt two masses in his abdomen. He'd hadn't felt any pain or bulge in the area, but an ultrasound revealed that besides a brain tumor, Philip had **polycystic kidney disease** (PCK).

This one-two punch rocked Philip to his core. He knew of no history of PCK disease in his family—quite unusual, though the disease sometimes skips generations or may have manifested itself in a relative who died without knowing they had the condition. At the time, Philip's kidney function was normal, often the case in PCK detected early. Abnormal function may not appear until the age of 40 or 50.

First things first, doctors successfully removed Philip's tumor. So much for problem number one. The struggle with problem number two, however, was just beginning.

In 2000, I saw Philip for a renal consult. He'd been reading about PCK and was anxious about possible kidney failure and winding up on dialysis. His creatinine was 1.8, suggesting about 40% loss of kidney function. He exhibited mild hypertension but otherwise felt well.

I explained that if we controlled his blood pressure, replaced Vitamin D early, controlled his phosphorous level with diet and observed him closely, he could work, play, and travel. We'd keep a steady eye on lab results, so if they suddenly tanked we could pursue a preemptive kidney transplant before he needed dialysis.

Philip had two sisters, both willing potential donors. One sister made it very clear to Philip that when the time came for a transplant, she wanted to be "the one."

Sisterly love, plain and simple, no strings attached.

I followed Philip closely for several years, emphasizing perfect blood pressure control. During this period, he exhibited no PCK-related complications, like ruptured cysts with bleeding, abdominal pain, or infection. He remained on high alert, however, especially when the trend in kidney-function markers began indicating disease progression. His anxiety rose proportional to his rising creatinine.

Polycystic kidneys can grow to enormous size in some patients, and Philip was one of them. He watched helplessly as the girth of his abdomen grew, a constant reminder of diminishing kidney function, impending need for a transplant, and the increasing burden on his sister.

In 2003, Philip's two sisters were tissue-typed for potential kidney donation. Though early in the transplant "work-up," it comforted Philip to know a plan was in the works to whip kidney disease and restore normalcy to his life.

By late 2006, Philip's creatinine had climbed to 3.8, reflecting a 75% loss of renal function. His kidneys continued to grow, to a point where he could barely buckle his belt. Despite losing so much renal function, intact (hard-working) nephrons compensated for those not working, and Philip remained asymptomatic. Still, it wouldn't be long before he would evidence the fatigue and malaise of kidney disease.

Philip's sister Carol, who lived in Los Angeles, was the most vociferous early-on about giving him a kidney. Turns out, she was the best match as well. A married professional with children, she remained undeterred in her desire to bail out her brother.

In January 2007, Cedars Sinai accepted Philip for a kidney transplant with his donor sister. He remained quite concerned, however, because his polycystic kidneys would be left in place and likely continue to grow. The potential for bleeding, infection, and abdominal pain would remain.

Meanwhile, he learned that the University of Maryland had developed a procedure to remove polycystic kidneys while simultaneously transplanting a new kidney—a long, complex surgery entailing more risk but offering a chance to live without bulging, diseased organs.

In August, Philip consulted with doctors at the University of Maryland. Deemed suitable for the double procedure, he underwent surgery soon after, his grossly enlarged polycystic kidneys removed and replaced by Carol's beautiful, healthy kidney. To the transplant team's delight, urine flowed immediately.

I saw Philip immediately upon his return from Maryland, one of many frequent visits to follow, to closely monitor him during critical post-operative months, when rejection and infection are more likely.

But none of that happened. Philip's kidney function stabilized, with a creatinine of 1.5. His blood pressure remained normal. Surgical incisions healed without complication. Philip relished putting on his pants without a struggle. But most of all, he gushed with gratitude and love for his sister, who recovered quickly and returned to her vigorous life of parent, wife, and professional.

Still, Philip faced several challenges over the next few years.

The University of Maryland discharged Philip on two potent immunosuppressant drugs, Prograf and Myfortic. Prednisone, a steroid often prescribed for transplant patients (for life), was not prescribed because the transplant team believed the good match with his sister made it possible to avoid this drug and its side effects.

In May 2008, Philip's creatinine unexpectedly jumped from his baseline of 1.5 to 2.8, creating severe anxiety for him and that sickening feeling I always experience with a patient in trouble.

Imaging of the kidney ruled out any mechanical, surgically induced problem. A renal biopsy suggested rejection. Phil's blood pressure, which was already high, went higher. I couldn't promise we could reverse the process, but told him we very often can. We administered high-dose steroids and increased levels of the anti-rejection drugs he was already taking. Thankfully, Philp's kidney function returned to normal.

As with so many transplant patients, there were still challenges to navigate, often resulting from a compromised immune system. Philip's kidney function remained stable, but he developed frequent skin infections and sinusitis. I checked his immunoglobulin levels, which indicated he was deficient in IgG, an important source of an infection-fighting antibody. Also, IgG can stabilize kidney function in transplant patients. Philip has been on monthly IgG, maintaining a normal level. He suffers fewer infections and his improved kidney function remains stable to this day.

Philip has worked hard in his profession and enjoyed success. Now, he's slowly pulling back from the pressure of crunching numbers, meeting deadlines, and satisfying clients. More active and healthy than he's been in years, Philip is "back in the game." But, for a change, he's in control. The ball no longer plays him. He's plays the ball.

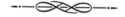

Chapter 10

Ashley

John Somics returned home a changed man after 18 months of horrendous military action in the jungles of Vietnam. He'd witnessed buddies bloodied, burned, wounded, and killed during ferocious combat with the Viet Cong. He suffered nightmares for months—relentless, terrifying visions of what he'd endured. So vivid were his dreams, John often awoke soaked in sweat, his pulse racing so fast he had to gasp for breath. Often, it took hours to return to sleep.

He was suffering a quintessential, clinical manifestation of stress.

Though supported by his parents after moving in with them in Santa Barbara, John never received much-needed professional emotional help. He was not particularly attuned to psychological issues and had received scant advice from the military about what to expect or how he might react upon reentering civilian life. In his mind, he would put his head down, his game-face on, "man up," and overcome his near-relentless anxiety. That was the toughness they'd taught him in the military. Surely it would work in civilian life.

John threw himself into his work in the construction industry, which was booming. He hoped work would help him forget the horrors of war, while he simultaneously built a new life, including independence from his parents. Over time, the nightmares occurred less frequently, but when they visited, he again awoke in a cold sweat, frightened, heart racing. Realizing they were dreams, he'd fall back on his pillow, eyes still riveted on the ceiling, but relieved that he lay in his own bed, not the muddy jungles of Vietnam.

Still, deep inside, he lived under constant stress, the current term for which is Post-Traumatic Stress Syndrome (PTSD). It's not new. It's been termed a lot of things in the past—shell shock, battle fatigue, and more. But no matter what you call it, PTSD can cause insurmountable stress and enduring physical and psychological harm. It can also lead to destructive habits to distract the mind, mute the pain.

John began drinking heavily and smoking cigarettes. At age 27, he met Tori, 25. She was warm, beautiful, and easy to be with. They married a year later.

Ashley, their middle daughter, told me this story of her parents and her childhood: At first, on the surface anyway, everything seemed fine in her parents' relationship, but they did not really know enough about each other to have entered a lifelong commitment. Their relationship was based more on appearances and less on passion, beliefs, or common goals for the future. Initially, Ashely said, her father kept his haunting demons a secret from the family. Later, she summed up her parents' relationship this way: An American vet, wounded so deeply that few could imagine his injury, and his young, naïve wife who had no idea of what was to come.

With the help of extended family, they bought a two-bedroom home in Santa Barbara. At first, John worked hard building homes while Tori began a career in the food industry. Then, suddenly, and without really discussing it, they decided to have children. Ashley's mother told her some years later that it just seemed to them that children followed marriage and their presence would be a tonic for a brewing troubled marriage. And if one child was good, they thought, three would be that much better. Elizabeth, Ashley's older sister, and Sean, her younger brother, completed the family.

It wasn't long until their parents' relationship began swirling in turbulence that emerges when a married couple can't express their feelings, fears, and frustrations, or lean on each other for support. Money woes added to the stress. John increasingly drank more to self-medicate his internal horrors while failing to aggressively seek work or bring home a steady paycheck.

Still, they had three children to support. Ashley's mother worked when she could, but she was the primary parent and felt compelled to stay home as much as possible with the children. As Ashely grew older, her respect for her mother grew. How her mom was simultaneously able to work and raise the children nearly by herself amazed her. Her father worked when work was readily available, but according to the children, he didn't vigorously pursue opportunities.

As Ashley grew up, finances continued pressing down on the family. Raising three children in Santa Barbara is expensive, and the Somics endured constant, immutable stress. Adding to the turmoil, they realized they needed more living space. Two bedrooms simply weren't enough for a family of five.

To John's credit, he planned to use his skills as a builder to remodel their home with the help of a friend. Unfortunately, financial planning to accomplish the task was flawed, plus John was ill-equipped to understand that his health was now at great risk due to his self-destructive lifestyle and the unrelenting stress from unresolved, unspoken internal conflicts.

The remodel began with adding a bedroom, but included plans for bathroom remodel and work on the kitchen. Ashley was in fifth grade when the project started. The remodel resulted in additional stress and took all of John's attention, effectively removing him from his young family. Making a bad situation worse, during the remodel Santa Barbara suffered severe winter storms that brought flooding and high winds. One night during a ferocious tempest, winds gusted to 70 miles per hour, blowing off their roof. Rain poured into the home, causing severe damage. Miraculously, nobody was injured, but instead of drawing the family closer, the event added even more stress, more straw to the proverbial camel's back.

The Somics moved into a small mobile home until the roof was replaced and the interior damage repaired. The remodel project seemed endless, delayed for weeks at a time due to lack of funds. The children were growing up quickly while John and Tori steadily grew apart.

Then, for no obvious reason, young Sean voraciously began drinking water and other liquids. He also complained about urinating more often and was clearly losing weight. A few months prior, he had suffered a severe viral upper respiratory infection, but nobody was overly concerned because he recovered routinely and only missed one day of school.

A pediatrician examined Sean after listening carefully to his history. He already knew Sean suffered from type 1 diabetes, or juvenile diabetes. His story was textbook for the disease: an upper respiratory infection predating the onset of diabetes. Once again, we observe: prolonged stress, followed by a viral infection and then manifesting as an autoimmune disease like juvenile diabetes.

The virus was likely the foreign invading protein that stimulated Sean's immune system, already weakened by significant family dysfunction, to allow immune complexes to attack his pancreas, rendering it unable to make insulin, resulting in juvenile diabetes. In a different person, with a unique genome and immune system, the same sequence might have resulted in lupus or some other immunologic illness. Clare, whose story I told earlier, suffered severe stress during her tumultuous divorce and simultaneous financial, job-related crisis. She developed a "flu-like illness" followed by a bizarre immunologic disease that destroyed her kidneys and nearly did the same to her lungs. It seems a spectrum of diseases manifest differently, but often have similar precursors—stress and infection.

In Ashley's already-besieged family, the level of tension, sadness, and stress now ratcheted up even more. Hospitalizations that Sean required early-on, associated with trying to balance his blood sugar using injectable insulin, terrified the entire family. Now, during this pandemonium, Ashley's mother had to learn to cook and prepare special sugar-free foods. Over time, Sean stabilized, gained weight and began to understand that a low-sugar diet and insulin injections were permanent accessories to his life. He accepted that, the remodeling of the house advanced more smoothly, and, for a short time, life all-around seemed better.

When Ashley entered 7th grade, she fell in love with running. Lean and healthy, she found it relieved the stress she'd been living with, leaving her mind refreshed. But, characteristically for Ashley's young life, nothing remained the same for long. Unexpectedly, during a track meet, she was unable to finish a mile run due to fatigue. Over time, she developed joint pain and generalized swelling. Her weakness progressed, her appetite decreased, and then she had a seizure. She was tested as UCLA, where results showed she had a positive ANA, consistent with systemic lupus. Blood tests also indicated she was in kidney failure. A renal biopsy revealed lupus nephritis, but due to the severity of damage to her glomeruli, treatment would unlikely reverse it.

Ashley was bewildered, confused, and devastated. In a short time, she'd gone from easily running several miles, to barely walking 100 feet without wilting under insufferable fatigue. She went from promising athlete to very sick patient in blink.

Despite long odds of successful treatment, UCLA opted to administer high doses of corticosteroids and CellCept, a drug targeting the immune system. Unfortunately, her kidneys did not respond. Making matters worse, her parents finally caved under the stress and separated, an event Ashley said was inevitable. For the children, the situation could not have been more difficult. Each suffered from the existing chaos, plus health problems that struck Ashley and Sean made the nightmare worse. Stress rained down upon the children and their parents, who finally divorced.

If this saga sounds strangely familiar, then you likely read Sarah's story. Both Sarah and Ashley endured relentless stress because their respective parents were incompatible. Moreover, anger the parents felt toward one another was not hidden from the children. In the end, even Ashley's parents had begun to use loud, aggressive words, aimed like darts, stinging the other, causing only more pain and anger. Both Ashley and Sarah (Chapter 3) were highly vulnerable 13-year-olds, just beginning adolescence, living in harsh environments. Both developed systemic lupus, accompanied by kidney failure.

Ashley's lupus didn't display usual signs like facial rash or joint swelling. It focused all its insidious, pathological fury on one organ system, her kidneys. When it reached a critical mass of renal destruction, Ashley had a seizure. Blood tests at UCLA revealed she'd lost complete kidney function, and that uremia caused the seizure that landed her in the Emergency Room.

Though emotionally stunned, having lost her ability to run, her kidney function, the unity of two parents for support, and any semblance of control over her life, Ashley instinctively knew she had to fight to survive. Tough sledding for a 13-year-old kid, but a kid with an iron will. Step one: life-saving hemodialysis to stabilize her tenuous medical condition. At UCLA, doctors placed a catheter in a large vein beneath her collarbone (you've read about this procedure, right?), then a series of dialysis treatments over a period of weeks restored metabolic balance and remove liters of excess fluid her body had retained. Finally, she began feeling better.

Still, after Ashley began outpatient hemodialysis, she cried most nights. This certainly wasn't what she imagined for her teenage years. She deeply missed exercise, her wellspring of emotional balance. Of course, she also endured harsh food and fluid restrictions. She continued taking powerful immunosuppressant drugs, which played havoc with her mood, though they did stabilize the systemic lupus.

By any measure, she was living a nightmare.

Ashley's mom, much like Sarah's mom, stepped up immediately to offer her daughter a kidney. It sounds like an easy thing that just rolls off the tongue or onto the printed page like no big deal. But, while it's a safe procedure for donors, it's an enormous life-changing event for recipient and donor alike. Ashley's mother successfully went through mandatory screening then donated her kidney to her daughter. Ashley left UCLA one week later with excellent kidney function. Her mother was medically fine and emotionally happier and stronger than she'd been in a long time.

With her new kidney functioning well, Ashley soon graduated from high school and ultimately went to college and studied to become a teacher. Her life and career went smoothly for many years. Her earlier medical challenges made her grateful for every day of good health. Finally, though, after sixteen years of stable kidney function, her healthy life fell apart again. Protein appeared in her urine, accompanied by some loss of kidney function. Shockingly, an ultrasound of her transplanted kidney showed a mass in its lower pole.

A biopsy of the mass revealed a papillary carcinoma, a low-grade cancer of the kidney. Both Ashley and her mother were crushed. Even though doctors explained that the cancer was an incidental finding that had nothing to do with the dysfunction seen in the gifted kidney, Tori felt guilty for having given her daughter a "flawed organ."

By now, you know the immune system's responsibility for destroying random cancer cells that, from time to time, enter our systems. The propensity for cancer may have been inherent in Tori and originated in her kidney. Ashley's immune system, beaten down by systemic lupus, chronic stress, and immunosuppressant drugs she'd taken since childhood, potentiated the growth of the cancer. For the same reasons, perhaps the cancer resulted de novo (on its own) due to a very compromised immune system.

Crushed by the diagnosis, Ashley had no choice but to have the cancerous kidney removed. In January 2016, Ashley underwent a transplant nephrectomy. The tumor was completely removed, but Ashley was left without a functioning kidney. She again found herself on that medical bus. Next stop, peritoneal dialysis.

Then, a longtime friend came forward to donate her kidney, again demonstrating everything noble in the human spirit. Ashley, of course, was incredibly grateful.

Even though immunologic compatibility between donor and recipient was poor, they utilized UCLA's paired donor program, which made an excellent match available from a donor in Colorado. The transplant scheduled, Ashley grew nervous and excited. A couple of days before the planned operation, however, she developed a high fever and pneumonia. She was hospitalized and treated for a fungal infection caused by pneumocystis, a rare disease seen almost exclusively in immune compromised patients, which if not treated early and aggressively, is quite dangerous and potentially lethal. Doctors treated Ashely with an antibiotic called septra, plus IVIG, and weeks later she was again ready for the paired-exchange transplant, which she received in September 2016.

Today, Ashley thrives. She's teaching again, and her passion to help dialysis patients has given her a great project to pursue. She has started a nonprofit corporation called, "Get Loud for Kidneys." Her organization will provide emotional support for kidney patients who need it to survive the kind of ordeal she endured.

Her mother is deeply relieved, happy for Ashley, and she, too, continues to stay healthy. Thoroughly examined, she remains cancer-free, including in her lone remaining kidney. Ashley's father, however, has developed type 2 diabetes and is struggling to control his disease. The theme that unabated stress, especially when coupled with mind-numbing self-medication like alcohol or addictive foods frequently causes adult onset diabetes, cannot be overstated because with early intervention, it's preventable. We'll talk more about that later.

Meanwhile, concludes, Ashley, "Considering where I've been and where I am right now, I'm extremely happy. My experiences have given me a deep understanding of what people with kidney problems face and I'm thrilled to be able to help them, as others helped me. What I've learned through all of this is that in the end, life is about what you can do for others."

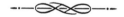

Chapter 11

Richard and Celeste

I first met Celeste when she was Director of Nursing for the Intensive Care Unit at Cottage Hospital in Santa Barbara. I remember being struck by her name—how beautiful and appropriate. Angelic in attitude, she nurtured relationships with patients in a heavenly manner that helped them heal.

One of few African Americans in a primarily white and Hispanic community, Celeste treated everyone equally, with love and compassion. She always impressed me with her thirst for teaching and excellence, but another quality, her ability to calm patients through honed listening skills and sensitivity to their plights, really caught my attention.

Celeste's own story of how she and her husband Richard courageously battled to provide him the highest quality of life despite his raging diabetes, and how they succeeded, makes her dedication to other patients even more profound. You could begin her story in a dozen different places, but perhaps starting at the unlikely moment she and Richard met would be best.

It began when Richard was at home one evening in Santa Barbara. He suddenly felt faint. Soon, he was shaking and incredibly weak. He called 9-1-1 just before slipping into shock. Paramedics found him on his living-room couch, delirious, hypotensive (low blood pressure), burning with fever. Concerned for his life, they inserted an intravenous line and began administering fluids. They lifted him onto a gurney, placed it in an ambulance, its siren screaming, and raced to Cottage Hospital.

The emergency room entrance resembled an episode from the television show, M.A.S.H. Paramedics pulled him from the ambulance, and with nurses and aides on all sides, rushed him inside within seconds. They administered more IV fluids to battle his low blood pressure and a severely infected wound. Doctors sent several blood cultures, a wound culture, and myriad tubes of blood to the laboratory to gain full understanding of his illness and its consequences.

Before long, Richard went from emergency room to the hospital's intensive care unit. There, as he struggled for life, Celeste entered the room. Then, of course, he was just a new patient, but to Celeste everyone deserved the best care and she was actively involved with all new arrivals. She walked quickly over and touched the back of his hand as he looked into her eyes. She told him he was going to be okay. She was especially convincing because something told her that Richard had a special reason to live. Turned out, she was right.

For over a decade before he met Celeste, Richard had worked in the small, south-central California town of Lompoc. An engineer, he kept a local hospital's technical apparatus up and humming. He was a deeply spiritual and religious man, married and devoted to his wife and his work. Life in Lompoc, was quiet and he was happy until the day his wife was diagnosed with advanced cancer. It spread quickly, far more quickly than Richard could emotionally absorb. Even his strong beliefs couldn't alleviate Richard's profound sadness and anxiety as the course of her cancer, despite chemotherapy and surgery, slid relentlessly downhill.

When it grew apparent that nothing could arrest the onslaught of his wife's cancer, and as Richard watched her fade, his anguish increased, and his spirits fell. His diet declined in step with his mental state. He began eating junk food and processed food every day, in large part because they were quick and easy to prepare, affording him more time to spend with his wife. He drank sugary sodas. French fries became a "food staple." Not only was this kind of food readily available, something about fried and sugary foods seemed comforting. What he didn't realize was that it was anything but comforting to his body. He gained lots of weight, but the damage was really being done inside his body, and his kidneys would be the ultimate victims.

When his wife passed away, Richard was mentally and physically devastated. Stress, of course, can have deadly effects, and coupled with his junk-food diet, his health was straddling the tracks of an oncoming freight train. Not long after his wife's funeral, he noticed something strange happening. He was relentlessly thirsty, and he constantly had to urinate. He began to lose weight, but not in a good way, and often felt dizzy. Later, he would learn the dizziness was caused by a blood-pressure drop, plus dehydration. All he knew then, however, was that he often felt wobbly, especially whenever he stood up. It scared him, so he checked in with his doctor, whose face grew serious when Richard described his symptoms. Even before he drew Richard's blood for sampling, the doctor said he believed Richard was suffering from new-onset diabetes. Richard had no idea what that meant. Over the next decade, however, he would learn all about it, as the disease played an increasingly major role in his life. A couple of days later, after that initial doctor's visit, tests came back confirming that Richard had slipped from the ranks of the "temporarily well." Like other patients described in this book, he then took his place on the perpetually moving medical conveyor belt, locked in the queue with no clue where it was headed.

At Cottage Hospital, Celeste read Richard's charts and saw he suffered from diabetes and resultant kidney disease. She also noted that he had undergone a successful kidney transplant a few years earlier. Unfortunately, it appeared that his diabetes was finally winning its war against the new kidney. Doctors ordered a large central line, called a Swan Ganz Catheter, to be placed into his subclavian vein and threaded through the right side of his heart, into the smallest pulmonary artery. Celeste knew he was very likely septic and would require careful monitoring of his cardiopulmonary pressures. The Swan Ganz would make this possible. Doctors delivered nasal oxygen, and measurements of pressures in his left atrium and pulmonary artery were taken while antibiotics went to work on bacteria hell-bent on destroying his entire body.

Richard's nephrologist arrived at the ICU to work with an intensive-care specialist. Lab results soon revealed Richard had an acute renal injury superimposed on his already faltering transplant. The intensive-care physician and a nephrologist concluded that a nasty recurrence of his diabetes was indeed attacking his transplanted kidney. A renal biopsy confirmed the diagnosis. Richard's charts revealed that in the past two years, he had experienced the well-documented, progressive complications from severe diabetes, the disease attacking his eyes, peripheral arteries, nerves, and heart. His severe infection had further damaged the kidney.

I was asked to take over Richard's care during his ICU admission. His kidney function, borderline before the event with a creatinine level of 2.2, was now seriously impaired.

Richard was highly immunosuppressed due to protocols required after his first transplant. During the first several years of his newly acquired kidney, he suffered several severe viral infections. He also had developed a nephrotic syndrome which, you'll recall, presented as massive loss of protein in the urine and swelling of the extremities. He lost important immunoglobulins in his urine, so he was hyper-vulnerable to infection. We talked openly about the future. He already knew severe infections and periods of very low blood pressure were often responsible for acute renal injuries. This he had suffered for sure, but could it be reversed? The consequences of one approach, drastically reducing or eliminating his immunosuppressive drugs, would be failure of his transplanted kidney and a return to dialysis.

Over the next few days, Richard's condition improved enough that he was transferred to a room on a medical floor. He was weak, depressed, and exhausted, but Celeste's daily visits inspired him and lifted his spirits. She offered soft, constant, comforting messages of hope. Their conversations soon ranged beyond Richard's medical issues. They shared funny stories of their childhoods and had long talks about spirituality. Turns out, they had similar religious beliefs, pillars of both their lives. A friendship blossomed, then something more emerged—a profound love for each other. Richard continued to recover under Celeste's watchful, loving eye, and they kept seeing each other after he left the hospital. Celeste was happy as a care-giver and Richard was thrilled to find love after ten years of being alone. They became inseparable.

During their many evenings together, they sometimes talked about the pathology of Richard's kidney disease. They both knew that extreme stress is one of the biggest killers on the planet, and that Richard had not been able to get through his wife's death without suffering enormous emotional downfalls. (As you'll learn later in this book, stress and poor eating habits likely trigger all manner of immunologic diseases, including rheumatoid arthritis, psoriatic arthritis, even systemic lupus. Still other, more common outcomes, may be a deep-dive into destructive lifestyle habits and/or the unmasking of latent diabetes.)

Celeste and Richard's relationship flourished, but, unfortunately, so did his diabetes. His recovery was not without great cost to his general health and wellbeing. His transplanted kidney continued to fail to the point where he returned to dialysis.

Out of that journey into darkness, however, entered light. He and Celeste grew increasingly serious about sharing a future together. She was in love with his courage and spiritual strength. He felt her faith and took great comfort from her presence. Soon, Richard proposed, and Celeste emphatically said, "Yes."

Love trumps diabetes every time.

Celeste recalls their wedding with great fondness. She told me that she and Richard laughed afterward about the priest asking her, "Do you accept Richard in sickness and in health?"—a question, of course, that had already been answered.

Richard required time to recover from the ordeal he had survived before even considering a second kidney transplant. He chose peritoneal dialysis and his engineering skills helped him master the procedure. He also now had his own personal nurse to watch over him.

Dialysis, however, was not the couple's biggest hurdle. It was, instead, the relentless onslaught of diabetes, which marches to its own drummer—difficult to control and associated with progressive disease of small and large blood vessels feeding the body's extremities. Richard, for one, began experiencing intermittent claudication (pain) in his legs, induced by walking. Atherosclerotic material composed of cholesterol and calcium began accumulating in his leg arteries, especially in his left leg. He felt subtle discomfort in his fingers, which would turn into something far worse over time.

During their first year of marriage, Richard's left-leg pain grew intractable. An angiogram revealed not only severe narrowing of a large blood vessel supplying his left leg, but evidence indicated small blood vessels had become occluded as well. Doctors attempted an angioplasty to dilate the affected blood vessel, but it proved ineffective. Unfortunately, occluded small blood vessels are untreatable. This forced Richard to undergo a below-the-knee amputation of his left leg. With Celeste behind him, and relying on their devotion to God, Richard courageously moved on, acquiring a prosthetic leg. With the help pf physical therapy, he learned to get around quite easily with it.

Then, Celeste announced something she had been considering for a few weeks. She could not stand to see her husband suffer any longer and decided she would gift her kidney to Richard. Urged on by Celeste, he decided to take the risk because life presently was so harsh for him. A functioning transplant seemed like a much better alternative.

Celeste knew Richard would be at risk for life-threatening infections and early loss of the kidney (due to his diabetes and post-transplant immunosuppression), but remained willing to do whatever she could to improve her husband's quality of life. She understood well that proceeding with a renal transplant was incredibly dicey, but her love and devotion carried Celeste forward, intent on seeing her husband thrive and enjoy life, even if for a short time.

To qualify for the transplant, Richard required a cardiac evaluation. An adenosine-thallium scan revealed three vessel diseases, which were successfully treated with the placement of three stents in critically narrowed coronary vessels. Clinging to their faith and love, they overcame this first series of hurdles. On to step two. Richard and Celeste shared the same blood type, and Celeste's health was perfect. Check. Step three: Interviews with a psychiatrist cleared Celeste as a donor, fully aware of risks involved and able to accept the consequences.

In 1998, the transplant took place at Cedars Sinai Hospital in Los Angeles—a joyous success. As kidney patients know, the best sign that things went well is when urine flows. It's not sexy, but it bring tears for even the toughest kidney transplant patients—donors and recipients alike. Celeste and Richard held hands and celebrated their triumphant moment. They both recovered without complication and within ten days went home to Santa Barbara.

I felt joy for them, but in the pit of my stomach a gnawing, uncomfortable feeling persisted, a feeling that reminded me of the potential for a treacherous course ahead. While they basked in results of the operation, I went to work figuring out how to maintain perfect blood sugar, blood pressure, and level of powerful anti-rejection drugs, the latter of which, while necessary to maintain transplant function, also bore the unfortunate side effect of making diabetes even more difficult to control.

In the time ahead, the biggest and most dangerous problem confronting Richard was the malignant nature of his diabetes. Even with Celeste's help and Richard's own commitment to maintaining a strict diet, metabolic balance proved impossible. Richard and Celeste suffered excessive stress, but they handled it with incomparable grace. Still, his cortisol level, a great indicator of stress, remained elevated all day, every day—a serious adversary counteracting the health benefits of insulin, making more difficult his efforts to control blood-sugar levels.

For several months, Richard's kidney functioned well, but toward the end of his first year post-transplant, protein appeared in his urine, quantities of which gradually increased from that moment on. The vascular component of Richard's disease worsened, leading to painful ischemic fingers (the result of diminished blood supply). Three fingers became severely painful and discolored. Surgery on the sympathetic nerves, called a sympathectomy, proved unsuccessful at relieving the pain. Finally, the three fingers were amputated.

One day, Richard noticed swelling in his normal leg. When I saw him in the office I asked if his urine looked like soap suds. He said yes. I knew immediately that he likely had developed the nephrotic syndrome, since foamy urine is a sign of heavy proteinuria. Tests confirmed my suspicion. During all of this, Richard and Celeste took each body-blow with courage and grace. They always sought solutions and didn't allow each other to show depression.

Over the next several months, they were severely taxed, emotionally and physically, due to recurrent, painful lesions in the tips of his remaining fingers. I used every remedy available to improve the blood supply to his fingers, without success. Richard requested my permission to try a specific mixture of Chinese herbs created by a highly respected doctor of Chinese medicine. I knew of the doctor, did some further investigations and in the end, I believed Richard was compliantly careful to use safe herbs that he obtained from China—he knew how to mix them in an ancient manner that served people well before the era of modern (Western) medicine. I had nothing better to offer, so I gave him my blessings.

For the next several months, Richard's hands improved slightly. Unfortunately, his kidney function deteriorated. News of this development, coupled with chronic pain, exponentially increased his stress level, making blood-sugar control still more difficult. Just like another subject in this book, Henry Murillo, who enjoyed a well-functioning kidney after his transplant, but ultimately succumbed to complications of diabetes, Richard was now on the same path, moving inexorably and inevitably toward the end. Though aware of his tenuous condition, he and Celeste never stopped enjoying all life had to offer. In fact, Richard's condition made them even more grateful for the time they had together. Celeste often said kidney disease drew them together and allowed them to spend the best times of their lives with each other.

Richard's heart began to fail, leading to a diagnostic coronary angiogram. It became clear he had developed (inoperable) diffuse, small-vessel coronary disease. Nothing could be done except to use anti-angina drugs while maintaining optimal blood pressure. He and Celeste spent one more sacred week together before Richard quietly passed away.

Though intensely sad, Celeste remained grateful for two things. First, Richard's physical pain had finally ended. Far more important, however, she knew they were blessed to have time together, full of loving moments, spiritual fulfillment, and joyous connections. For eight years, they lived a life of complete togetherness, fully aware that there's no guarantee anyone will get even six months of such a celestial connection.

Was Richard's fierce struggle, despite physical pain, diabetes, and other physical problems worth it? Celeste had no doubt that it was. Emotional and spiritual rewards had been immense for both, and Celeste knew Richard's indomitable spirit would live on through her and others he touched, including me.

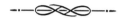

Chapter 12

Renal Transplantation

"It is when you give of yourself that you truly give."
--Kahlil Gibran

Clearly, a successful kidney transplant remains the ultimate therapy for ESRD patients. Receiving and maintaining a successful transplant, however, isn't simple. It can be a lengthy process, requiring a cast of special characters acting in harmony to make it happen.

When a kidney transplant succeeds, it generally follows a protracted drama—a long night's journey into day.

Act One begins with an unsuspecting patient living a normal life, unaware that a stealthy, silent disease is slowly destroying his or her kidneys. One day, the patient doesn't feel so well, or has a routine physical exam, then boom—a doctor tells them their kidneys are on the ropes. Basically, without serious intervention like dialysis, it's a death sentence. Typically, no matter how the message is delivered, shock and fear grip the patient, often numbing their ability to absorb this horrible news.

Act Two starts with life-restoring dialysis and the gift of time. Essential groundwork begins here, decelerating a patient's anxieties and establishing trust in the doctor who will shepherd them through illness and help navigate rough waters ahead. Early referral from a primary-care physician to a nephrologist (the moment lab work indicates renal dysfunction) provides more time for patients to absorb the news and rationally plan their future. It also facilitates a smoother transition to dialysis and transplantation.

(Unfortunately, many patients, especially the undereducated and poor, don't have the luxury of early diagnosis. They often wind up in the ER with symptoms of complete kidney failure before seeing a nephrologist. Many are African American or Latino, suffering hypertension, diabetes, obesity, heart disease, and high cholesterol—the "metabolic syndrome.")

The Final Act, either before dialysis even begins or following an intermission of dialysis lasting months or years, features a kidney transplant—a notion so profound, so surreal, it begs an array of questions, like, "How can we remove a kidney from one person and surgically place it in another with confidence it will function?" or, "Who thought of transplanting an organ into another human being in the first place? And, "How did the science of transplantation evolve?" Also, commonly, "What is life like for a patient dependent on another's kidney?" and, "How does the life of a living donor change?"

For answers, let's start with a "transplantation timeline."

The concept is certainly not new. Indian physician Sushruta considered it 2,500 years ago. Although he never transferred an organ from one being into another, he developed devices to reconstruct amputated noses and earlobes. He published his results in 500 BC, in Sushruta Samhita, his medico-surgical compendium.

In 1902, Austrian surgeon Emerich Ullmann performed the first kidney transplant, placing a dog's kidney into the neck of another dog. It lasted five days. In 1906, German surgeon Ernst Unger transplanted a pair of monkey kidneys into the thigh of a girl dying of kidney failure. They failed to produce urine. Nonetheless, the following year Simon Flexner, a medical researcher at the University of Chicago, predicted it would someday be possible to substitute a healthy organ like a kidney for a diseased one.

He was correct, but it would take time.

In 1933, a Russian surgeon transplanted a kidney, removed six hours earlier from a deceased donor, into the thigh of a patient dying from uremia. Their blood types were incompatible, so it rejected almost immediately.

A giant leap forward came in 1950, when Ruth Tucker, a 44-year-old with PKD, received a kidney transplant that functioned for ten months before failing. At the time, very little was known about the immune system's role and the importance of tissue compatibility in renal transplants. Moreover, immunosuppressant drugs didn't yet exist.

In the 1950's, a group of pioneering French surgeons known as the "French Transplantation Club" performed several kidney transplants. Although the transplants failed because of immune incompatibility, the operations broke new surgical ground. The kidneys were placed in the pelvis of recipients, outside the peritoneal membrane—the procedure of choice to this day.

An important milestone, maybe the most important, was achieved in 1954 at Peter Bent Brigham hospital in Boston, where transplant surgeon Dr. Joseph Murray and nephrologist Dr. John Merrill transplanted a kidney from one identical twin to the other. It functioned immediately and lasted eight years. From this success, the modern science of immunology was born, as scientists began studying mechanisms of compatibility that allowed a genetically identical donor and recipient to thrive.

At the UCLA Medical Center in 1960, corticosteroids were used for preventing organ rejection. Next came the development of **azathioprine** (a.k.a. Imuran), used together with steroids to treat diseases of an overly aggressive immune system like Lupus, and to prevent renal transplant rejection.

Using these two drugs, results began improving, ushering in the modern age of kidney transplantation. In the process, we learned that each of us has an immune system that deploys when a foreign protein, such as a viral infection, invades our body. Unique cells called B cells (special lymphocytes in our blood) recognize a foreign invader and quickly kill it. This "immune surveillance" protects us from infections as well as cancer cells.

Unfortunately, it also mobilizes against transplants.

Because donor-kidney cells contain specific biological markers (antigens) absent in a recipient's cells, the transplanted kidney looks like a foreign invader, signaling the recipient's immune system to make antibodies to destroy (reject) it. The human immune system simply can't discern between a lifesaving transplant and a life-threatening infection.

Studying nephrology in 1972, I witnessed kidney-transplant patients frequently reject their new organs. Placed on high-dose corticosteroids to help reverse the process, they often suffered terrible complications, including deadly infections. Clearly, we were still in the Dark Ages of transplant science.

During my training at UCLA, Dr. Paul Terasaki, a distinguished professor of surgery and immunology, was developing a test that would become the international standard for tissue typing. This procedure, which assesses the compatibility of organ donors and recipients, has been used for kidney, heart, liver, pancreas, lung, and bone-marrow transplants for the past 40 years. His work dramatically reduced morbidity from transplant malfunction and led to stunning improvements in transplant success.

Dr. Terasaki's discovery of histocompatibility antigens, or **Human Leukocyte Antigens (HLA)**, define "match compatibility" between donor and recipient. Only six of these antigens are needed to evaluate compatibility. These six come in more than 100 forms not equally present in the human population. The most common HLA antigens are present in only 20% of us, plus some HLA antigens provide a stronger immune response than others. These variables can make finding a compatible donor other than a family member difficult. When a family member matches with all six antigens, we called it a "full house."

Scientists, however, have developed techniques to "fool" the immune system into not only allowing non-family-member transplants, but allowing an unrelated recipient with an incompatible blood type (by current standards a poor genetic match) an excellent shot at success. New, superior drugs suppress the immune system more selectively, while plasmapheresis, discussed earlier, "softens the immunological beachhead," further enabling chances for normal kidney function.

Today a full house is welcome, but not essential for success.

We also have "paired kidney donations" (discussed earlier)—an algorithmic advance, which, married to sophisticated tissue-typing, allows doctors to "pluck" pairs of donors and recipients from a pool of living-transplant "participants" for the best possible outcomes, bypassing the need for direct, binary compatibility. This way, a donor's kidney may go to a stranger, but still results in a successful transplant for a friend or loved one.

Before a transplant can occur, however, prospective donor and recipient must undergo vigorous testing to be sure they qualify. Both are screened for cancer, infections such as AIDS or hepatitis, heart disease, pulmonary disease, and psychological competency. For the recipient, immunosuppressant drugs can cause a tiny cancer to spread quickly. If an infection is present, it could become life threatening. In the presence of emotional issues, steroids and other meds can wreak havoc with the patient's ability to handle stress.

The donor, moreover, must be in great health with two normal kidneys. In addition, they must willingly want to give the gift of life. Wishy-washy won't do. Trained screeners also look for any sign that a donor was coerced or promised recompense, monetary or otherwise.

Furthermore, donors must be prepared for failure. They are instructed, more than once, that the transplant might fail, and are asked if they would consider that a personal failure. This task and others falls to mental-health experts on the "work-up team."

Surgeons typically remove the gift-giver's kidney using a laparoscope—a fiber optic instrument inserted into the abdomen. They remove the kidney through a small incision in the same region—far less painful than the "old way," which required a large surgical incision under the donor's backside ribs, plus a longer postoperative recovery. Today, most donors are home in 3-5 days and back to work in a few weeks.

The donor receives ongoing medical care to confirm good kidney function and rule out post-surgical complications. If the donor was carefully screened and follows a prevention and wellness routine moving forward, there appears to be little risk. (Some studies even suggest slightly increased longevity for kidney donors compared to the general population, often attributed to increased health awareness. Transplantation, however, hasn't been around long enough to definitively confirm this.)

For the recipient, Act One of a second drama has just begun. They leave the hospital on a metabolic high, with a functioning transplant and a new regimen of powerful drugs intended to protect it from rejection, most common during the first 4-6 months.

Still, some 10-40% of transplant recipients experience an acute rejection episode during the first six months post-transplant, most often successfully treated by increased doses of immunosuppressant drugs. Eventually, the doses are reduced to safer levels. Toward the sixth to eighth year post-transplant, though sooner in some cases, previously undetectable **donor-specific antibodies (DSAs)** may cause transplant function loss and ultimately lead to kidney failure. These days, physicians usually maintain doses of immunosuppressant drugs at higher levels than in the past, to prevent this. Meanwhile, the world's top transplant researchers and physicians continue pursuing the goal of eliminating this vexing problem of "chronic rejection" altogether.

Still, even chronic rejection doesn't necessarily mean the end of good kidney function. Some patients, including several in this book, lose their transplant after many years of healthy life, then move on to a second, third, even fourth kidney. Mick, for example, enjoys excellent health with his fourth transplant.

(Here's added good news: New assays can now detect immunoglobulin G (IgG) antibodies. A recent study at Yale showed that transplant recipients who had a specific positive IgG antibody, a DSA. were six times more likely to lose their kidneys than those who did not. More frequent renal transplant biopsies, looking for subtle abnormalities such as micro protein in the urine or a very small rise in creatinine, plus immunologic testing for DSA, may help us prevent kidney loss by applying plasmapheresis and increasing doses of immune-system blocking drugs. The cellular and immunologic biology of rejection is much better understood now, leading to increased transplant graft survival.)

New transplant patients take antiviral, anti-fungal, and anti-bacterial medication for the first several months, to prevent commonly acquired infections. The transplant team sees these patients frequently, twice-weekly at first, then weekly, monthly, quarterly, semiannually, and, finally, sometimes, just once a year. Using sophisticated analytic tools, they vigilantly watch for even the subtlest signs of rejection, so they can treat them immediately.

More good news: newer immunosuppressant drugs, induction therapies to remove dangerous antibodies that could attack a new kidney, and paired matching programs have made transplants safer and more effective than ever. The danger of severe infections or malignancies is much lower than in the past, though common side-effects like basil-cell and squamous-cell skin cancers remain common.

Thirty years ago, an increase in temperature might have caused concern about an exotic infection gaining foothold in an immunosuppressed patient. Today, it's more likely a common cold or viral infection. That said, any blood test showing a small increase in serum creatinine or a urinalysis detecting any protein raises concern about infection or rejection, including possible return of the patient's original kidney disease.

This leads to new tests, possibly including a biopsy, and, of course, terrifies the patient. Again, in the modern era of transplantation, serious, irreversible "acute" rejections are quite rare and the duration of good kidney function far exceeds what it was in the "old days," when I was a renal fellow.

And the patient's job? They need to "own" their new kidney, dutifully take their medication, and submit to routine blood draws that allow doctors to measure (and adjust as necessary) immunosuppressant-drug levels. They need to eat right, exercise and rest, especially patients who were previously diabetic or prone to diabetes, due to the ironic fact that the very medicines that help prevent rejection can also cause diabetes and can decrease kidney function in the new transplant ("nephrotoxicity").

Transplant recipients also need to embrace the notion that every day is glorious, borrowed time. The worst thing a patient can do is think, "I feel great, so I'll stop taking my meds because they must have done the trick." That mindset paves the road to rejection and back to dialysis. And trust me, transplant teams are reluctant to try again with non-compliant patients. They consider them an excessive risk and a potential waste of time, money, and precious, limited resources—human kidneys.

And for anyone on dialysis with a transplant from a relative in the works, it's likely you'll do well for a long period. In fact, all transplants are functioning better and longer than they did just 10 years ago. Donors, universally, are thriving with no adverse consequences from their generous gifts.

The final byproduct of increasingly successful kidney transplants is, of course, love. Donors and recipients draw close and stay close for years, fused by altruism and gratitude, angled ever-closer to the real meaning of life.

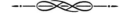

Capítulo 12

Trasplante Renal

Claramente, un trasplante de riñón exitoso sigue siendo la terapia definitiva para los pacientes con insuficiencia renal. Recibir y mantener un trasplante exitoso, sin embargo, no es tan simple. Puede ser un proceso largo y extenso, que requiere de un elenco de personajes especiales, actuando en harmonía para que esto ocurra.

Cuando un trasplante de riñón tiene éxito, generalmente sigue un curso ensayado — un viaje nocturno largo hacia el amanecer.

El primer Acto comienza con un paciente que lleva una vida sana, sin saber que una enfermedad sigilosa, silenciosa está lentamente destruyendo sus riñones. Un día, el paciente no se siente tan bien, o tiene un examen físico rutinario, entonces sopas!, un médico les dice que sus riñones están contra las cuerdas. Básicamente, sin una intervención seria, es una sentencia de muerte. Por lo general, no importa cómo es entregado el mensaje, ira y miedo se apoderan del paciente lo cual adormecen su capacidad de absorber esta horrible noticia.

Acto dos comienza con el tratamiento de diálisis y esperar que pase el tiempo. Es en esta etapa donde el grupo de diálisis se esfuerza en disminuir ese estado de ansiada y establecer esa confianza para poder ayudar al apaciente a navegar por aguas turbulentas más adelante. Es primordial que en cuanto se descubra inicios de problemas renales, el paciente sea referido a un nefrólogo para una evaluación mas detallada. Esto nos da tiempo de planear su futuro medico. Al mismo tiempo, esto también facilita una transición menos estresante a la diálisis y al trasplante.

(Desafortunadamente, muchos pacientes, especialmente los que están bajos de educación y de bajos ingresos, no tienen el lujo de saber un diagnostico a tiempo. Muy a menudo terminan en la sala de urgencias con síntomas de insuficiencia renal muy avanzada antes de ver a un nefrólogo. Muchos son afroamericanos o latinos, padeciendo de hipertensión, diabetes, obesidad, enfermedades del corazón y colesterol alto, lo que viene siendo un «síndrome metabólico».)

El acto final, antes de que comience la diálisis o después de una interrupción de la diálisis con duración de meses o años, es un trasplante de riñón, una noción tan profunda, tan surrealista, que pide una serie de preguntas, como, "¿Cómo podemos quitar un riñón de una persona y colocar quirúrgicamente en otro con la confianza que funcionara?" o "quien iba pensar en trasplantar un órgano a otro ser humano en primer lugar? Y, "Como es que la ciencia del trasplante haya evolucionado?" Además, y comúnmente, "¿Cómo es la vida de un paciente de trasplante de riñón?" y, "¿cómo es la vida de un donante de riñón?"

Para responder estas preguntas, vamos a empezar con una " línea de tiempo sobre el trasplante."

El concepto ciertamente no es nuevo. Un médico indio Sushruta consideró un trasplante hace 2,500 años. Aunque él nunca trasplantó un órgano de una persona a otro, él desarrolló dispositivos para reconstrucción de lóbulos de las orejas y narices amputadas. Él publicó sus resultados en el ano 500 A.C., en el Sushruta Samhita, su compendio medico-quirúrgica.

En 1902, cirujano austríaco Emerich Ullmann realizó el primer trasplante de riñón, colocar el riñón de un perro en el cuello de otro perro. Este duró cinco días. En 1906, un cirujano alemán Ernst Unger transplanto un par de riñones de mono en el muslo de una niña que se estaba muriendo de insuficiencia renal. Estos fallaron puesto que no producian orina. Sin embargo, al año siguiente Simón Flexner, un investigador médico en la Universidad de Chicago, predijo que algún día sería posible sustituir un órgano sano por un riñón de un enfermo. Él estaba absolutamente correcto, pero tomaría tiempo.

En 1933, un cirujano ruso trasplanto un riñón, este riñón se había obtenido 6 horas antes de que la persona hubiera fallecido, en el muslo de un paciente muriendo de uremia. Sus tipos de sangre eran incompatibles, por lo que su rechazó fue inmediato.

Un enorme paso adelante llegó en 1950, cuando Ruth Tucker (44 anos) recibió un trasplante de riñón que funciono por 10 meses antes de que fallara de nuevo. En aquel entonces, se sabia muy poco sobre el papel del sistema inmune y la importancia de la compatibilidad de tejido en trasplantes renales. Por otra parte, no existían todavía medicamentos inmunosupresores.

En la década de 1950 un grupo de pioneros cirujanos francés conocidos como el "Club de trasplante francés" realiza varios riñón trasplantes. Aunque los trasplantes fallaron debido a la incompatibilidad inmunológica, las operaciones abrieron nuevos caminos quirúrgico. Los riñones se colocaron en la parte pélvica de los beneficiarios, fuera de la membrana peritoneal, este hasta la fecha es el procedimiento preferido.

Un punto importante, tal vez el más importante, ocurrió en 1954 en el hospital Peter Bent Brigham en Boston, donde el Dr. Joseph Murray y nefrólogo Dr. John Merrill trasplantó un riñón de un gemelo idéntico a otro. Funcionó inmediatamente y duró ocho años. De este éxito, la moderna ciencia de la inmunología nació, los científicos comenzaron a estudiar mecanismos de compatibilidad que un donante genéticamente idéntico y recipiente para que estos prosperaban.

En el centro medico de UCLA en1960, se utilizaron corticosteroides para la prevención de rechazo de órganos. Luego vino el desarrollo de la **azatioprina** (también conocido como Imuran), utilizado junto con esteroides para el tratamiento de enfermedades de un sistema inmune demasiado agresivo como el Lupus y para prevenir el rechazo de trasplante renal.

Con estas dos medicinas, los resultados comenzaron a mejorar, marcando el comienzo de la era moderna del trasplante de riñón. En el proceso, aprendimos que cada uno de nosotros tiene un sistema inmune que despliega cuando una proteína extraña, como una infección viral, invade nuestro cuerpo. Únicas células llamadas células B (linfocitos especiales en nuestra sangre) reconocen al invasor extraño y a rápidamente acaban con él. Esta "vigilancia inmune" nos protege de infecciones, así como las células cancerosas.

Por desgracia, esto también ataca contra los trasplantes.

Porque las células de riñón de donantes contienen marcadores biológicos específicos (antígenos) ausentes en las células del receptor, el riñón trasplantado mira como un invasor exterior, avisándole al sistema inmune del receptor a hacer anticuerpos para destruirlo (rechazarlo). El sistema inmunológico humano simplemente no puede discernir entre un trasplante y una infección potencialmente mortal.

Cuando estudiaba Nefrología en 1972, fui testigo de como muchos trasplantes rechazaban sus nuevos órganos. Estos pacientes eran puestos en altas dosis de corticosteroides para ayudar prevenir el rechazo, pero a menudo esto causaba terribles complicaciones, incluyendo infecciones mortales. Claramente, en ese entonces estábamos muy ignorantes de la ciencia del trasplante.

Durante mi entrenamiento en UCLA, el Dr. Paul Terasaki, un distinguido profesor de la cirugía y la inmunología, estaba desarrollando una prueba que se convertiría en el estándar internacional para la tipificación del tejido. Este procedimiento, que evalúa la compatibilidad de órganos donantes y receptores, se ha utilizado para el riñón, corazón, hígado, páncreas, pulmón, y los trasplantes de médula ósea por los últimos 40 años. Su trabajo ha dramáticamente reducida morbilidad de mal funcionamiento del trasplante y conducido a impresionantes mejoras en el éxito del trasplante.

El descubrimiento de Dr. Terasaki de antígenos de histocompatibilidad o **Antígenos de leucocitos humanos** (HLA), definir el "partido de compatibilidad" entre donante y receptor. Sólo seis de estos antígenos son necesarios para evaluar la compatibilidad. Estos seis vienen en más de 100 formas y estos no están igualmente presentes en la población humana. Los antígenos HLA más comunes están presentes en sólo el 20% de nosotros, y algunos antígenos HLA proporcionan una respuesta inmune más fuerte que otros. Estas variables pueden hacer difícil a un donante compatible que no sea un miembro de la familia. Cuando un miembro de la familia coincide con todos los seis antígenos, le llamamos un " suertudo".

Sin embargo, los científicos han desarrollado técnicas para "engañar" al sistema inmunológico en hacerlo aceptar no nomas trasplantes a gente con parentesco biológico pero en aceptar trasplantes a personas sin ningún parentesco, sin ninguna compatibilidad sanguínea y con una exitosa compatibilidad. Ahora, tenemos medicamentos mas superiores que supriman el sistema inmune en una forma más selectivamente, mientras la plasmaféresis, la cual discutimos anteriormente, "suaviza todo el sistema inmunológico para que sea mas dócil", lo cual hace que el riñón sea mas aceptado por el cuerpo y funcione mejor.

Hoy cualquier riñón es bueno, pero no tiene que ser 100% compatible para que trabaje.

También existe un programa llamado " intercambió de riñones" el cual fue discutido anteriormente), donde un método algorítmico, computa por medio de datos clínicos ala mejor pareja de compatibilidad medica sin tener que someterse a pruebas medicas directas. Esto permite que un trasplante de riñón puede ir a una persona completamente extraña, mientras el donante del paciente puede donarle su riñón a otra persona que sea lo mas compatible posible.

Antes de un trasplante pueda ocurrir, sin embargo, el posible donante y receptor deben someterse a vigorosas pruebas medicas para asegurarse que los dos están clínicamente capacitados para tal procedimiento. Ambos son revisados clínicamente buscando enfermedades como cáncer, infecciones como el SIDA o hepatitis, cardiopatía, enfermedad pulmonar y trastornos psicológicos. Esto es muy importante porque para el receptor, los medicamentos inmunosupresores pueden despertar células cancerosas que rápidamente se riegen y se multipliquen. Si una infección está presente, esto podría llegar a ser algo mortal. En presencia de problemas emocionales, los esteroides y otros medicamentos pueden causar que el paciente pierda los estragos y la capacidad para manejar una crisis emocional.

El donante, por otra parte, debe estar en buena salud con dos riñones normales. Además, deben voluntariamente *querer donar o regalar* este regalo de vida. El hecho de que nomas se ofrecen de lengua sin que deveras lo hagan, no vale nada. Inspectores clinicos capacitados en esta materia, también buscan cualquier señal si la persona fue presionada, o prometida alguna recompensa, monetaria o de otra manera.

Además, los donantes deben estar preparados para lo peor, como un fracaso. Ellos son instruidos, más de una vez, que el trasplante puede fallar y se preguntó si consideran que un fracaso personal. Por esta razón, los consejeros mentales se aseguran que la persona se someta a una prueba psicológica para poder encarar cualquier fracaso.

Cirujanos normalmente quitan el riñón del donador usando un laparoscopia (un instrumento de fibra óptica) que se inserta en el abdomen. Quitan el riñón a través de una pequeña incisión en la misma región, un procedimiento mucho menos doloroso que el "antes", que requeria una incisión quirúrgica grande debajo de las costillas de parte trasera del donante, además de una recuperación postoperatoria más larga. Hoy, la mayoría de los donantes están en casa en 3-5 días y regresan a trabajar en un par de semanas.

El donante recibe atención médica constante para confirmar que su riñón funcione bien y descartar posible complicaciones post quirúrgicas. Si el donador se evalúa con cuidado y sigue una rutina de prevención y bienestar para el resto de su vida, es muy seguro que sus riesgos sean minimos. (Algunos estudios sugieren incluso ligeramente mayor longevidad para los donadores de riñón en comparación con la población en general, quizás por mejor empeño en el cuidado personal de la salud. Como la ciencia del trasplante es una área relativamente nueva, lo acabado de mencionar no se puede confirmar definitivamente.

Para el paciente del trasplante, una nueva hazaña acaba de empezar. Es muy común que salgan del hospital con un alto metabolismo, con un nuevo trasplante y un nuevo régimen de medicinas potentes destinadas a proteger y prevenir un rechazo, lo cual es más común durante los primeros 4-6 meses.

Aun con las mejores medicinas, existe un 10-40% de pacientes que sufren un episodio de rechazo agudo durante los primeros seis meses, el cual es tratado aumentando trató con éxito aumentando la dosis de medicamentos inmunosupresores. Conforme el paciente acepte el nuevo riñón, las dosis de medicinas se reducen a niveles más seguros. Hacia el sexto o octavo año pos trasplante, y a veces en muchos casos, previamente indetectables anticuerpos específicos de donante (**DSA**) puede causar pérdida de la función del trasplante y en última instancia conducen a insuficiencia renal. Estos días, los médicos suelen mantener la dosis de medicinas inmunosupresores a niveles más altos que en el pasado, para evitar esto. Mientras tanto, lideres en esta rama continúan inventando tratamientos médicos para que el dia de mañana se elimine por completo el "rechazo de riñón crónico".

Aún así, rechazo crónico incluso no significa necesariamente el final de la función renal . Algunos pacientes, incluyendo varios en este libro, perdieron su trasplante después de muchos años de vida saludable, siguieron con el segundo, tercero e incluso cuarto riñón. Mick, por ejemplo, goza de excelente salud con su cuarto trasplante.

A pesar de todo de todo esto, hay buenas noticias en el horizonte. Se esta trabajando con nuevos ensayos de sangre que logran detectar los anticuerpos inmunoglobulina G (IgG). Un estudio reciente de la Universidad Yale demostró que los pacientes de trasplante tenían un anticuerpo IgG positivo específico, un DSA. Estos pacientes son seis veces más propensos a perder sus riñones que aquellos que no lo tienen. El hecho de poder hacer biopsias de trasplante renal más frecuentes, en busca de anormalidades sutiles como micro proteínas en la orina o un muy pequeño aumento en creatinina, además de pruebas inmunológicas para DSA, nos pueden ayudar a prevenir pérdida del riñón haciendo la plasmaféresis y aumentando la dosis de medicinas bloqueadoras de sistema inmune. En la actualidad, la biología celular e inmunológica de rechazo se entiende mucho mejor ahora, conduciendo a una aumento del trasplante de la supervivencia del trasplante.

Es muy común que pacientes con nuevo trasplante tomen medicamentos antivirales, contra hongos y medicamentos contra bacteria por los primeros meses, evitar y prevenir infecciones comunes. El equipo de trasplante ve a estos pacientes con frecuencia, dos veces por semana al principio, luego semanal, mensual, trimestral, semestral y, finalmente, a veces sólo una vez al año. Utilizando sofisticadas herramientas analíticas, vigilan y miran con mucho cuidado cualquier inicio de rechazo, y tratarlo inmediatamente.

Más buenas noticias: nuevas medicinas inmunosupresoras , terapias de inducción para eliminar anticuerpos peligrosos que podrían atacar un riñón nuevo y programas de intercambio han hecho trasplantes más seguro y más eficaces que nunca. El peligro de infecciones graves o neoplasias malignas es mucho menor que en el pasado, aunque los efectos secundarios comunes como cánceres de piel de siguen siendo una amenaza.

Treinta años antes, un aumento de temperatura corporal hubiera sido algo preocupante en un paciente con bajas defensas. Hoy en día, lo miramos como un resfriado común o una infección viral. Dicho esto, cualquier examen de sangre que muestre cualquier aumento en la creatinina tan pequeño q sea o un análisis de orina demostrando cualquier cantidad de proteína eleva preocupación por infección o rechazo, incluyendo el posible regreso de la nefropatía o la enfermedad original del paciente.

Esto conduce a nuevas pruebas sanguíneas, posiblemente incluyendo una biopsia y, por supuesto, esto es aterrador hacia el paciente. Una vez más, en la era moderna del trasplante, los rechazos serios y irreversibles son absolutamente raros y la duración de la función renal del paciente supera la calidad de vida comparada con los "viejos tiempos" cuando apenas yo era un novato de medicina.

¿Y cual es el trabajo del paciente? Que crean en su nuevo riñón, que sean "dueños" de su nuevo riñón, que se tomen las medicinas diario y religiosamente y que se sometan a chequeos de sangre rutinariamente que nos permita (nosotros los médicos) medir (y ajustar si es necesario) los niveles del sus medicinas. Los pacientes tienen que aprender a comer una dieta balanceada, hacer ejercicio continuo y regularmente, especialmente los pacientes previamente clasificados diabéticos o propensos a la diabetes, debido al hecho irónico de que los mismos medicamentos que ayudan a prevenir el rechazo también pueden causar diabetes y pueden disminuir la función renal en el trasplante nuevo "(lo que se llama una intoxicación nefrotoxica).

Los pacientes de trasplante también tienen que valorar la idea de que cada día es una bendición y que nuestro tiempo en esta vida es limitado o prestado. Lo peor que puede hacer un paciente es pensar, "Me siento muy bien, así que voy a dejar de tomar mis medicamentos porque ya paso la tormenta y ya me siento bien". Esa mentalidad conduce al camino del rechazo y para atrás a la diálisis. Y créanme, los centros de trasplantes se niegan a trasplantar otra vez si saben que el paciente perdió el trasplante for falta de incumpliendo al programa de medicinas. Esto es considerado como un riesgo excesivo, una pérdida de tiempo, dinero y otros recursos valiosos, limitados — como son los riñones humanos.

Y para cualquier persona en diálisis con un trasplante de un familiar en proceso, es probable que su cuerpo lo acepte por mucho tiempo. De hecho, todos los trasplantes en la actualidad están funcionando mejor a comparación de mas de 10 años.

El resultado final de trasplantes de riñón cada vez más acertado es, por supuesto, amor, mucho amor. Donadores y receptores se mantienen en constante contacto por muchos años, ligados por el altruismo y la gratitud, lo cual es un ángulo grandioso que le da un verdadero sentido a la vida.

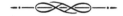

Chapter 13

How to Get a Kidney Transplant

"He who has the why to live for can bear almost any how."
--Fredrick Nietzsche

Walking, talking, seeing, hearing, digesting, breathing, sleeping. We take most bodily functions for granted until something goes haywire. Same goes for urinating, with one big exception. You can still pee when something goes wrong, very wrong, with your kidneys. You just don't know it until these forgiving organs slip below 30% function, by which time it's often too late to save them. And without kidney function, or a sustaining substitute like dialysis, life is not possible.

Below 30% function, you'll begin feeling crappy, with any number of symptoms, like nausea, muscle cramps, swollen ankles, diminished appetite, fatigue, or sleeplessness. You head to the doctor, who'll typically begin with family history and a physical exam. Your physical may appear normal, with the likely exception of high blood pressure and maybe a little protein in your urine. Next come blood tests and a urinalysis.

Then the first bombshell falls and your emotional roof collapses.

Reviewing lab results, the doctor explains that your kidneys are failing. Following more tests, maybe a renal biopsy, a more definitive diagnosis emerges and you're told bad news and good, usually in that order. The bad news: Your kidney disease is irreversible and you'll soon need dialysis. The good news: You're likely a candidate for transplantation. That's where the "Transplant Tutorial" begins.

Step One: Remain calm.

When you first learn how sick you are and the potentially dire outcome of your illness, a cyclone of anxiety, along with a dizzying array of information, may overwhelm you. That's okay, and it's very normal. You'll have time to digest it all and learn about the life-altering and life-saving path forward. This is going to be a long journey—months, maybe years—but you can't complete it if you don't start, and that begins now.

The first step is straightforward. Don't panic. Stay calm, keep it together. If you don't, rational thinking diminishes and the temptation to emotionally dissolve or "give yourself over to fate" may erode your will to persevere. Breathing exercises help. Deep breaths, in through the nose, out through the mouth. Deep breathing and the calm it generates will help you focus, listen, absorb information, and plan for challenges ahead. Repeat these exercises several times a day.

Don't isolate yourself. Talk to family members, loved ones and friends about your situation. Building a support network is the first pillar of a team effort that's key to adapting to life-change and getting a new kidney. It may also send an early message to someone—family member, friend, colleague, roommate—who may wind up being a donor. But don't advance that notion now; it's way too early for you and them (it will make them nervous and emotionally conflicted). Just knowing you're sick is enough information for now. There's plenty of time ahead to assess the landscape of options for you and people who care about you.

Step Two: Keep all appointments with your doctor and come prepared.

Never miss a doctor's appointment. This is vitally important, especially early in your odyssey, when what you don't know far exceeds what you do know. Come armed with questions, as physicians may be pressed for time and not know the precise nature of what concerns you most. Write down questions prior to an appointment, so you don't forget them. Come with an advocate—family, friend, colleague. They provide emotional support and can help you remember (or append) questions you may have.

Clear communication is especially important for non-English-speaking patients, particularly Hispanics, whose population bulges with kidney disease. Bring a bilingual interpreter to help ask questions and translate answers. Ask where you can get Spanish-language literature, and, on dialysis, request consistent communication with Spanish-speaking nurses, nutritionists and social workers (or people who can advance your questions and comments to somebody *who does* understand them).

Step Three: Make your intentions known.

Begin discussing transplantation with your doctor as soon as your health, confidence, and comfort allow. If they say, "Well, we'll talk about that down the line," tell them, "Yes, I know it won't happen tomorrow, but I want to start planning for it today."

The earlier you plant the seed, the better. That way, you send a clear message to your health-care team about your frame of mind and determination to beat kidney disease with the only therapy allowing a return to normal life. Tell them early-on and remind them often. Silence and acquiescence are your worst enemies. It takes time, effort, and team work for your doctor to shepherd you to a transplant. If they don't know that's your rock-solid goal, it's easier to "warehouse" you on dialysis— arguably the saddest outcome plaguing renal-disease therapy today.

Above all, remember this key for navigating the path forward, and repeat it to yourself often: Nobody cares more about you than you! Don't be shy. Don't worry about annoying doctors with questions. Don't worry about asking where you can get up-to-date information on dialysis and transplantation. It's your future at stake, nobody else's. Embrace this notion, from the time the doctor solemnly tells you your kidneys are failing to the moment they slide you onto the transplant operating table.

It can save your life.

Step Four: Educate yourself.

If you're on dialysis or headed there, learn about your disease, its effects, and your options to control it. Read patient literature on kidney disease, dialysis, and transplantation. You can find it at your doctor's office, dialysis unit, transplant center, or through the National Kidney Foundation. Online resources are abundant. Become an expert on you. Ask questions of everyone—nurses, doctors, nutritionists. You simply won't know the answers unless you ask, and health-care providers can't read your mind.

Join a kidney support group in your region. People with transplants or awaiting one exchange valuable information at group meetings that may help connect you with folks in similar situations or provide guidance on the "do's and don'ts" for getting a new kidney and maintaining it. You can find these groups through your dialysis center or closest transplant hospital.

Ask your doctor if they know kidney recipients who are willing to share their stories and tips for reaching your goal. They've gone through what you're going through and often have valuable guidance to offer. I have several transplant patients who volunteer these services.

Step Five: Lifestyle compliance.

Normally, dialysis initially makes you feel better—the so-called "honeymoon phase." But you will inevitably grow bored, even agitated, by depending on a machine to sustain you 9-12 hours a week. So bored and agitated, in fact, that you may slip into a dietary comfort zone, eating foods and drinking fluids that can harm or kill you. Don't do that. It can trigger a downward spiral that wrecks your health and your chances for a new kidney. Remember, this is a marathon, not a sprint.

Dialysis requires huge lifestyle adjustments, maybe the toughest you've ever faced. Nurses and nutritionists will explain the details and importance of taking your meds and adhering to a strict "renal diet" that includes limited intake of certain foods and severe fluid restrictions. Rigorously follow their advice. Take your meds every day and on time, including multiple pills required with meals. Avoiding foods you may love but will make you sick, and limiting fluid intake will test your mettle, but these are two necessities for nutritional compliance.

By complying, you'll feel better and tolerate dialysis better. The less fluid you drink, despite raging thirst, the less stress on your vascular system and the less fluid to eliminate on dialysis. "Squeezing" 10 pounds of fluid from a non-compliant patient in one dialysis session is not only a tricky, stressful challenge for nurses, it takes more time, leaving a patient drained, cramped, and miserable. Lifestyle non-compliance can also lead to stroke, heart attack, and death.

Another benefit of compliance relates to your kidney-transplant goal. Your dialysis charts contain information about every treatment you have: weight gained between treatments, weight removed on dialysis, hours of dialysis, blood chemistry, and more. So, while you're on dialysis at noon on a Monday, the health-care team—doctors, nurses, nutritionists, and social workers—are in a conference room reviewing patient files. They candidly discuss cases, especially tough ones the team is working on to gain compliance from non-compliant patients (non-compliance is not only hard on a patient, it's hard on care-givers tasked with muscling through that patient's resistance to provide humane, necessary care).

In fact non-compliance doesn't help your chance of getting a transplant, either. First, you may not be healthy enough to receive a cadaver kidney that comes available at 2:00 a.m. on a random Tuesday morning. Second, if you're non-compliant on dialysis, transplant centers are leery to risk your non-compliance with a new kidney, considering 70,000 other people in the U.S. are also waiting for one. In short, kidneys are too precious a resource to waste on non-compliant patients. Conversely, a compliant patient is not only ready for the 2:00 a.m. call, but they're "in the mix" to receive a kidney from a living donor. Summarized, compliance will make you feel better and help you get a kidney quicker.

Step Six: Finding a donor.

As soon as your health-care team, in coordination with your local transplant center, deems you an acceptable transplant candidate, they'll register (or "list") you with the Organ Procurement and Transplantation Network (OPTN), which maintains a centralized computer network linking all regional organ-gathering organizations and transplant centers. The United Network for Organ Sharing (UNOS), a private nonprofit organization, administers OPTN under a contract with the Federal Government.

You've come a long way, digested devastating health news, managed the shift to dialysis, complied with its regimen of lifestyle restrictions, informed yourself about your options, and now taken a big step toward receiving a new kidney. You're "listed."

Since waiting for a genetically compatible cadaver kidney can take months, often years, there's no need to sit around waiting for the renal version of the Publishers Clearing House to call.

So, go find your own kidney. You've already been deemed a suitable candidate, now it's on you to find a living donor to speed up the process. Many times, a family member will step up. They often make great donors, owing to genetic similarities to you. If you need a kidney, and they offer, accept it. I've had patients with healthy, willing family donors tell me, "I don't want to disrupt their lives," or "I couldn't accept a kidney from my own flesh and blood." And there they linger, often for years, awaiting a cadaver kidney that may arrive, may not.

Certainly, this is a matter of individual choice. But realistically, for a dialysis patient needing a kidney, your own flesh and blood is exactly what you need, exactly what will give you the best chance for a successful transplant that lasts many years. Plus, consider this: donors, especially family members, want to help because they love you. Why leave them frustrated or deny them the eternal satisfaction of rescuing you from that cliff from which you're dangling? Honestly, this is no time for martyrdom. If you get the chance, get out of that dialysis chair and get on with your life.

Let's assume, now, that you don't have family members either willing or able to donate. Then it's time to spread the word, because, thanks to breakthroughs in immunology and genetic matching, people not related to you can make great donors, too.

Start with the internet, email and Facebook, for example (and there are more social-media platforms). Think of all the people you know—

friends, colleagues, church group, college roommates, book club, bowling league—then get their email addresses and blast off a simple query. One patient, we'll call him Joe Smith, told me his strategy was not to ask for donors directly, but to have a friend or loved one send an email on his behalf. This was his version, written by his brother Bill:

Dear friends and family,

As you may know, my brother Joe has been on dialysis for some time and needs a kidney transplant. If you are interested in donating a kidney to Joe or know someone who might wish to donate, please contact him at xxx-xxx-xxxx. He can explain what's involved with giving "the gift of life." For more donor information, see https://www.cedars-sinai.edu/Patients/Programs-and-Services/Comprehensive-Transplant-Center/Kidney-and-Pancreas/Donating-an-Organ.aspx

Thanks for considering a kidney donation to Joe.

Sincerely,

Bill Smith

Simple, direct, not overly emotional, this approach offers two advantages:

First, when somebody sends a query on your behalf, it doesn't strike the recipient as a desperate plea, or, frankly, begging. It strikes them as a humane outreach by a friend or loved one on behalf of somebody else. It puts the email recipient at ease, allowing them the time and space necessary to digest the information, discuss it with others, and reply or not. Receiving an email directly from you might make them feel pressured and less likely to fully consider their options.

Second, it subtly encourages recipients to forward the message to other people who also forward the message, and so on. In this manner, you start a chain reaction that may result in kidney donation by a friend of a friend of a friend who you know only casually, maybe exchanging holiday cards once a year. I've seen this happen more than once. There are heroes out there, we just don't know who they are until times like this. And they often come from the most unexpected places. So, spread the word and remember, you are the master of your fate.

Now, let's say somebody steps up to offer you a kidney. This loving gesture, from whomever it comes, is always jaw-dropping. The first thing to do is talk with them, meet with them, take walks together if you live in the same town. This will not only begin sealing a special bond, it allows the two of you to discuss the life-saving importance of this potential gift and the process for delivering it.

Next comes the "work up" at your local transplant center. You and your potential donor will be evaluated separately. They will have blood tests, chest X-ray, psychological evaluation and more. If they're deemed fit and ready to move forward, the transplant team will set a surgery date. Before that day, you may be treated with pre-transplant infusions and plasmapheresis to reduce the chance of rejection.

On transplant day, you'll be wheeled into an operating room, where a team of experts—transplant surgeons, urological surgeons, highly trained nurses, anesthesiologists—are waiting for you and your donor kidney, the latter delivered by a similar team of experts in another room, on the "extraction" side of this double surgery.

You'll sleep for a few hours and wake up with a new kidney. You'll be blurry and dopey for a while, hooked to a jungle of machines, monitors, and tubes. Doctors and nurses will attend to you regularly. You'll feel like their top priority, their only priority. If the kidney has started working immediately—as they often do—doctors will inform you as your creatinine level steadily drops toward your ultimate baseline. Patients tell me that on about the third day post-transplant, they can feel wellness returning as their blood chemistry normalizes. For many, it brings buckets of tears to feel well for the first time in a long time.

Now, let's draw back from this perfect outcome and consider a different one. Suppose your potential donor, a friend, for example, doesn't match you well enough for a transplant. That's when you work with your doctor and transplant center to enter a paired-exchange program. Remember that process? That's when a pair of incompatible donors exchange kidneys with another pair of incompatible donors to transplant the most genetically compatible kidney into each recipient. Though recipients don't directly receive kidneys from their original, intended donors, all parties get what they want—donors donate and "their" recipients receive the gift of life.

Most transplant centers have their own paired-exchange programs, and there are national programs as well. Be sure to inquire about them and look them up on your own. As discussed earlier, paired exchange, while not an immunological breakthrough, has been one of the greatest advances in kidney transplantation in recent years.

There is, however, a caveat. Your initial prospective donor must agree to participate in a paired exchange program, knowing that they may never meet the person who receives their kidney, but at the same time their intended recipient will get one.

So, now you're listed for a cadaver transplant and you have a donor in the mix for a paired exchange. But why stop there? Other potential donors may connect with you, as well. Any one of them might be a good match, so repeat the same procedure you did with the first potential donor—work-ups and evaluation in coordination with your nephrologist and transplant center.

You may hit the jackpot with donor number two, and never look back. Or, donor number two may not match you but is also willing to enter the paired exchange program. I've had patients with several potential donors, all of whom agreed to participate in paired exchange, given opportunity and circumstance. As a recipient, that just increases your odds of receiving a kidney and receiving it faster.

So, remember: Don't panic, remain hopeful, communicate, educate yourself, make your intentions known, buckle in for a long ride, persevere, comply with a strict lifestyle regimen, get listed, and find a living donor.

That's how you get a kidney transplant

Capítulo *13*

Cómo Obtener Un Trasplante de Riñón

Caminar, hablar, ver, oír, digerir, respirar, dormir. Todo esto lo tomamos ala ligera hasta q algo deja de funcionar. Lo mismo va para orinar, con una gran excepción. Es muy común que auque podamos orinar, algo se encuentre mal, muy mal con los riñones. Simplemente, uno no se da cuenta que algo esta mal hasta que ya el 30% de esa función se ha perdido. A este punto, es muy difícil and corregir el problema de los riñones. Sin función renal o substituto como diálisis, la persona termina falleciendo.

Por debajo del 30% de la función renal, uno se empieza a sentir enfermo, con un sin número de síntomas, como náuseas, calambres, tobillos hinchados, disminución del apetito, fatiga o insomnio. Esto conduce ala persona a visitar a su medico quien toma el historial medico y hace un examen físico. Ojo!, el examen físico puede ser normal con la excepción de presión arterial alta y quizás trazos de proteína en la orina. Luego vienen los exámenes de sangre y un análisis de orina.

Al enterrarse de las anormalidades químicas, el primer bombazo cae y se viene una torrente de emociones inexplicables.

Al repasar los resultados de laboratorio, el médico explica porque los riñones están fallando. Después de más pruebas, incluyendo una biopsia renal, surge un diagnóstico más definitivo y se vienen malas y buenas noticias, generalmente en ese orden. La mala noticia: la enfermedad renal es irreversible y que pronto necesitará diálisis. La buena noticia y todo depende de varios factores: es probable que el paciente sea candidato para un trasplante de riñón.

Aquí es donde empieza el "Tutorial de trasplante".

Paso uno: mantener la calma.

Cuando uno aprende por primero lo grave de la enfermedad, se viene un ciclón de la ansiedad, junto con una gran cantidad y variedad de información, lo cual puede ser abrumadora. Esto es muy común y es completamente normal. Ya habrá tiempo para digerirlo todo y aprender mas sobre lo que se viene. Esto es el comienzo de un viaje largo, que se llevara meses, quizá años, pero uno no puede terminar si no ha empezado, se comienza hoy!

El primer paso es sencillo. No te asustes. Mantén la calma, no hay que alarmarse. Si uno se descontrola y pierde la calma emocional, es muy fácil inundarse en un remolino depresivo que simplemente impide que la persona persevere y pierda todo control emocional.

Los ejercicios de respiración aquí son fundamentales. Respiraciones profundas, a través de la nariz, y fuera por la boca. Respirando profundamente y manteniendo la calma generan ala persona a concentrarse mejor, escuchar, absorber información y planear para futuros desafíos. Es muy saludable que estos ejercicios se repitan varias veces al día.

No se aislade. Hable con sus familiares, seres queridos y amigos sobre su situación. Construir un equipo de apoyo es el primer pilar y clave para empezar la adaptación hacia un nuevo cambio de vida hasta que un trasplante de riñón sea disponible. También puede uno enviar un mensaje temprano a alguien, miembro de la familia, amigo, colega, compañero de piso, que puede terminar siendo un donante. Pero no se desespere, esta idea quizás empeore la situación creando mas ansiedad y emociones conflictivas. Sólo hágales saber que está enfermo y eso es suficiente información por ahora. Tenga la seguridad que habrá mucho tiempo para evaluar el panorama de opciones que estarán disponibles para usted y las personas que se preocupan por usted.

Paso dos: mantener todas las citas con su médico y venir preparado!

No se pierda ni una cita médica. Esto es vital, especialmente temprano en su odisea, es como cuando uno piensa que sabe mas de lo que en verdad uno sabe. Venga armado con muchas preguntas. Estos sumamente importante especialmente si el medico no sabe lo que mas le preocupa. Haga una lista de preguntas antes de la cita para que no se le olvide preguntarlas. Venga con una persona que abogue por usted, un familiar, un amigo, un colega. Alguien que pueda brindar ayudar emocional y le ayude a recordar preguntas que pueda tener.

Una comunicación clara es especialmente importante para los pacientes que no hablan inglés, especialmente los hispanos, cuya población sufre de mas enfermedad renal. Si puede traiga un intérprete bilingüe que ayude a hacer preguntas y respuestas de traducion. Pregunte donde puede conseguir literatura es español sobre la diálisis, hable con enfermeras que hablan español, nutricionistas y trabajadores sociales (o pida que sus preguntas sean referidas a personas que entiendan su situación).

Paso tres: Haga saber sus intenciones.

Comenzar a hablar de trasplante con su médico tan pronto como su salud, confianza y comodidad lo permitan. Si dicen, "Bueno, vamos a hablar sobre este tema mas adelante," entonces usted diga, "Sí, yo sé que esto no va a pasar mañana, pero quiero empezar a planear y planificar desde hoy."

Lo mas pronto que usted siembre esa semilla, mejor. Así, envía un mensaje claro a su equipo medico sobre su estado de ánimo y la determinación para vencer la enfermedad renal con la única terapia que permite una vida que le devolverá su normalidad. Dígales temprano y recuérdeles a menudo. Guardar silencio y no preguntar preguntas son sus peores errores que uno puede hacer. Recuerde que esto se toma tiempo, esfuerzo y trabajo para que su médico lo guie hasta que reciba un trasplante. Si su equipo renal no sabe cual es su meta real, es muy fácil que la persona se "almacené" en diálisis por mucho tiempo, desafortunadamente esto sucede muy a menudo en centros de diálisis.

Por eso, recuerde esta frase para navegar por el camino a seguir y repetirla a menudo a sí mismo: nadie se preocupa por mi mas que yo mismo! No sea tímido. No tienes porque preocuparte al preguntar muchas preguntas a los doctores. Si se molestan, que se molesten! Asegúrate de obtener información lo mas actualizada posible sobre la diálisis y trasplante.

Esta es tu vida y tu futuro es que esta en juego aquí, de nadie mas. Lucha y aprende los mas que se pueda sobre tu enfermedad desde el momento que te dicen que tus riñones están fallando hasta el dia que te ingresan al quirófano para un trasplante. Lucha! Lucha hasta el final. Esto puede salvar tu vida.

Paso cuatro: Edúcate.

Si estas en diálisis o vas empezar diálisis, aprende todo sobre la enfermedad, sus efectos y opciones para controlarla. Lea literatura sobre su enfermedad renal, diálisis y trasplante. Esta puede encontrarla en su consultorio de su doctor, unidad de diálisis, centro de trasplantes o a través de la Fundación Nacional del riñón (NKF, siglas en ingles). Hay mucha información y recursos en la internet. Buscala. Conviértete en experto en uno mismo. Hazle preguntas a todo el mundo, enfermeras, médicos, nutricionistas. Uno nunca va a saber las respuestas a muchas de sus preguntas a menos que pregunte, y entiendo que su equipo medico no le puede leer su mente. Pregúnteles!

Únete a un grupo de apoyo de riñón en su area. Estos grupos de apoyo facilitan la conexión entre personas con situaciones similares y puedan proporcionar información o consejos sobre el "Qué hacer y qué no hacer" para conseguir un riñón nuevo y como mantenerlo. Estos grupos se pueden encontrar en su centro de diálisis o centros de trasplantes. Pregunte.

Pregúntele a su doctor si saben de pacientes de riñón que están dispuestos a compartir sus historias y consejos para alcanzar tu meta. Pregunte. Esta gente han pasado por su misma situación y muy a menudo ofrecen muchos consejos valiosos en como en encarar su situación. Yo tengo varios pacientes de trasplante dispuestos a compartir sus historias.

Paso 5: cumplimiento de normas de estilo de vida.

Normalmente, diálisis al principio te hace sentir mejor — la llamada "fase de luna de miel." Pero inevitablemente se aburrira, se enojara, al darse cuenta que tiene que depender de una máquina de 9-12 horas a la semana para sobrevivir. Se aburrera o enojara tanto que quizás caiga en una zona de confort dieta, donde come alimentos y bebe líquidos que pueden dañarlo o hasta matarlo. No haga eso! Esto puede desencadenar un espiral descendente que arruinaría su salud y las posibilidades de obtener un nuevo riñón. Recuerde que esto es un maratón, no un sprint.

Diálisis requiere muchos ajustes en su vida, quizás estos sean los retos mas difíciles que va enfrentar. Su equipo de enfermeras y nutricionistas le explicará todos los detalles y la importancia de tomar sus medicamentos y adherirse a una estricta "dieta renal" que incluye limitaciones of ciertos alimentos y estrictas restricciones de líquidos. Siga sus instrucciones rigorosamente. Evite sus comidas preferidas, ya que estas puedan empeorar su enfermedad y limite la cantidad de fluidos que uno toma a diario. Esto ultimo es fundamental para que su salud lleve una dieta adecuada y se mantenga estable.

Cumpliendo con estas normas, uno se sentirá mejor y podrá tolerar mejor la diálisis. Entre menos líquido beba, a pesar de la maldita sed, esto será mas saludable para su sistema vascular y menos fluidos serian eliminados por la diálisis. "Exprimir" 10 libras de líquido de un paciente desobediente en una sesión de diálisis no es sólo un reto complicado y estresante para los enfermeros, pero se lleva más tiempo, dejando al paciente chupado, acalambrado y miserable. Al no seguir con sus indicaciones medicas, puede llevar a accidentes cerebrovasculares, ataque cardíaco y muerte.

Hay otro beneficio con la meta de obtener un trasplante de riñón. Su expediente de diálisis contienen información acerca de cada tratamiento: peso subido entre los tratamientos, peso quitado en diálisis, horas de tratamiento, laboratorios químicos y mucho más. Mientras que usted está reciviendo diálisis al mediodía de un lunes, el equipo de salud: médicos, enfermeras, nutricionistas y trabajadores sociales — se encuentran en una sala de conferencia repasando archivos clínicos de pacientes. Esta junta se enfoca en discutir caso por caso particular-mente casos de alto riesgo donde el paciente batalla con su enfermedad y requiere mas atención o cuidado del equipo de diálisis o de su apoyo familiar. La falta de responsabilidad personal del paciente complica que su estado clínico se mantenga estable. Esto es sumamente frustran-te para la familia y su equipo medico quienes ponen todo de su parte para que el paciente lleve una vida sana y estable.

De hecho, el no cooperar y no seguir el régimen de diálisis dis-minuye sus chanzas de conseguir un trasplante de riñón. En primer lugar, esto indica que la persona no pueda estar lo suficientemente sana o sano para recibir un transponte de riñón que muy común esta disponible als 2 d mañana en un martes ala azar. En segundo lugar, si eres desobediente con su programa diálisis, los centros de trasplante son muy cuidadosos en ofrece trasplantes de riñón a personas que no cumplen con sus responsabilidades medicas entendiendo que hay mas de 70,000 personas en los Estados Unidos esperando uno. En otras palabras, los riñones en la actualidad son unos órganos muy valiosos y se hace todo esfuerzo para que estos sean destinados para pacientes que deberás lo valoren y lo cuiden. Por el contrario, un pa-ciente obediente no sólo está preparado para la llamada de 2:00 de la mañana, pero están "en la mezcla" de pacientes para recibir un riñón de un donante vivo. En pocas palabras, cumpliendo con sus respons-abilidades medicas y estando estable aumenta sus probabilidades de obtener un rinon mas rápido.

Paso seis: encontrar un donante .

Tan pronto como su equipo de salud, en coordinación con su centro local de trasplantes, lo considera un candidato aceptable de trasplante, será registrado con la organización nacional llamada Organ Procure-ment and Transplantation Network (OPTN), la cual mantiene un ban-co de datos computarizados que están conectados a todas las organi-zaciones regionales de órganos y centros de trasplante. La red unida para compartir órganos (UNOS), es una organización privada sin fines de lu-cro, administra OPTN bajo un contrato con el Gobierno Federal.

Hasta ahora, usted ha recorrido un largo camino, digerido devastadoras noticias de salud, logró ajustarse ala diálisis, cumplir con su régimen de restricciones de estilo de vida, aprendió acerca de todas sus opciones sobre varios tratamientos de su enfermedad y ahora un paso mas para recibir un riñón nuevo. "Enlistado"

Ya que la espera de un riñón de cadáver genéticamente compatible puede tomar meses, años, no hay necesidad de esperar la llamada de la versión renal de los Publishers Clearing House.

Por lo tanto, manos a la obra, empecemos a buscar su propio riñón. Ya sabemos que paso todas las pruebas medicas y es candidato para un trasplante, entonces empecemos la búsqueda de un donante vivo para acelerar el proceso. Muchas veces, un miembro se conmueve y le ofrece un riñón. A menudo ellos son los mas compatibles genéticamente hablando. Si usted necesita un riñón, y le ofrecen uno, acéptelo!. He tenido pacientes con familiares dispuestos a donar y me dicen, "No quiero interrumpir su vida", o "No podía aceptar un riñón de mi propia carne y sangre." Y de ahí no salen, se pasan meses y a veces años, en espera de un riñón de cadáver que quizás llega, quizás no.

Sin duda, cada quien toma sus propias decisiones. Pero ya realmente hablando, si estas diálisis y necesitan un riñón, esto es *exactamente* lo que necesita, su propia carne y su propia sangre. Esto es *exactamente* lo que le daría la mejor oportunidad para que su trasplante sea exitoso y dure muchos años. Además, considere esto: los donantes, especialmente miembros de la familia, quieren ayudarlo porque lo quieren y lo estiman. ¿Por qué dejarlos frustrado o negarles la eterna satisfacción de rescatarlo de ese barranco de donde usted está colgado? Honestamente, este no es el momento para el martirio. Si tienes la oportunidad, tomala, y deja esa silla de diálisis, hágase el trasplante y viva su vida al máximo.

Supongamos, ahora, que no tiene familiares o amigos dispuestos a donar. Entonces es tiempo de difundir la voz, porque, gracias a los avances en Inmunología y genética que conjunta parejas, gente no relacionada con usted pueden ser buenos donantes también.

Comience con el internet, correo electrónico y Facebook, por ejemplo (y hay más plataformas de medios sociales). Piensa en todas las personas que conoces, amigos, colegas, grupo de la iglesia, compañeros de colegio, compañeros de boliche etc, entonces obtenga sus direcciones de correo electrónico y mándeles una simple invitación haciéndoles saber de sus necesidades.

Un paciente, lo vamos a llamar Joe Smith, me dijo que su estrategia fue no pedir por un rinon directamente, sino que un amigo o ser querido enviar un correo electrónico en su nombre. Esta fue su versión, escrita por su hermano Bill:

Queridos amigos y familia,

Como ustedes saben, mi hermano Joe ha estado en diálisis durante algún tiempo y necesita un trasplante de riñón. Si usted está interesado en donar un riñón a Joe o conoce a alguien que desee donar, por favor póngase en contacto con le en xxx-xxx-xxxx. Él puede explicale el proceso a seguir con tal regalo "el don de la vida". Para más información de donante, ver https://www.Cedars-Sinai.edu/patients/Programs-and-Services/Comprehensive-Transplant-Center/Kidney-and-pancreas/donating-an-Organ.aspx

Gracias por considerar una donación de riñón a Joe.

Atentamente,

Bill Smith

Simple, directo, no excesivamente emotivo, este enfoque ofrece dos ventajas:

En primer lugar, cuando alguien envía un mensaje asi de su parte, no suena como que la persona esta desesperada o que esta llorando a gritos. Al contrario, este mensaje suena como algo caritativo y de buena voluntad. Pone al destinatario del correo electrónico tranquilo, permitiendo tiempo y espacio necesario para digerir la información, discutirla con otros y responder o no. Recibir un correo electrónico directamente de usted podría hacerlos sentir con mas presión, causar ansiedad y ponerlos menos propensos a reconsiderar todas sus opciones.

En segundo lugar, muy sutilmente y subconscientemente, anima a los destinatarios para reenviar el mensaje a otras personas que también reenviar el mensaje y así sucesivamente. De esta manera, se inicia una reacción en cadena que puede resultar en donación de riñón de un amigo de un amigo de un amigo que conoce sólo por casualidad, tal vez nomas se intercambian tarjetas de Navidad una vez al año. He visto esto suceder más de una vez. Hay muchos héroes, simplemente uno no los conoce hasta momentos como estos. Y a menudo vienen de los lugares más insospechables. Por lo tanto, corra la voz, difúndala y recuerde, usted es el amo de su propio destino.

Ahora, supongamos que alguien se anima le ofrece un riñón. Este gesto amoroso, de quien sea que venga, siempre es algo asombroso. La primera cosa que tiene que hacer es hablar con ellos, reúnase con ellos, caminen juntos si viven en la misma ciudad. Esto no es sólo el comienzo de un comienzo de un sello especial, sino el comienzo de una relación encadenada que permitirá el tiempo de discutir la importancia de salvar una vida, y hablar de este regalo sagrado hasta mas allá de la cirugía.

A continuación siguen todos los "preparativos" en su centro local de trasplantes. Tú y tu posible donador se someterán a evaluaciones separadas. Tendrán exámenes de sangre, radiografía de tórax, evaluación psicológica y mucho más. Si todo sale en orden y no hay ningún impedimento, el equipo de trasplantes fije la fecha de cirugía. Antes de ese día, usted puede tratado con infusiones de pre-trasplante y plasmaféresis para reducir la posibilidad de rechazo.

En el día del trasplante, usted será llevado al quirófano, donde un equipo de expertos — trasplante cirujanos urológicos, cirujanos, anestesiólogos, enfermeros altamente capacitados, están a la espera de usted y su riñón, este último es entregado por un equipo similar de expertos en otra habitación, al lado de la "extracción" de esta cirugía doble.

Podrá dormir por unas horas y despertarse con un riñón nuevo. Vas a sentirse medio borracho y tonto por un rato, conectado a una gran cantidad de máquinas, monitores y tubos. Médicos y enfermeras lo asistirán regularmente. Te sentirás como su más grande prioridad, su única prioridad. Si el riñón ha empezado a trabajar inmediatamente, como lo hacen a menudo, los médicos le informará su nivel de creatinina desciende constantemente hacia su última línea de fondo. Muchos pacientes me dicen que como al tercer día pos trasplante, la persona empieza a notar la diferencia ya que sus niveles en la sangre se empiezan a normalizar. Para muchos, esto trae baldes de lágrimas al sentirse bien por primera vez en mucho tiempo.

Ahora, vamos a retroceder de este resultado perfecto y considerar uno diferente. Supongamos que el donador potencial, un amigo, por ejemplo, no es compatible lo suficientemente bien como para ser donador. Aquí es donde a su donador se le ofrece participar en un programa especial donde el donador se inscribe en un intercambio de riñones. ¿Recuerdas ese proceso? Es entonces cuando un par de riñones de donantes incompatibles se comparan con otro par de donantes incompatibles y se escoge el donante que es mas compatible con usted. Aunque los destinatarios directamente no reciben riñones de sus donantes originales, previstos, todas las partes consiguen lo que quieren — aquí todos ganan, los donantes donan y «sus» destinatarios reciben el regalo de vida.

La mayoría de centros de trasplante tiene sus propios programas de intercambio emparejado, y también hay los programas nacionales. Asegúrese de preguntar acerca de ellos e investigar más a fondo por su cuenta. Como lo comentamos anteriormente, el intercambio de riñones, aunque no es un avance inmunológico, ha sido uno de los mayores avances en el trasplante de riñones en los últimos años.

Sin embargo, hay una advertencia. Su posible donador debe estar de acuerdo en participar en un programa de intercambio emparejado de riñones, sabiendo que nunca podrán reunirse o conocer a la persona que recibe sus riñones, pero al mismo tiempo su destinatario recibirá uno.

Así que, ahora que ya está enlistado para un trasplante de cadáver y tienes un donante en la mezcla para un intercambio. Esto no es todo. Porque dejar las cosas hasta aquí? Otros posibles donadores pueden comunicarse con usted y ofrecerle un riñón. Cualquiera de ellos podría ser un buen donador, así que repita el mismo procedimiento que hizo con el primer donador potencial-Explíqueles los pasos a seguir para la evaluación en conjunto con sus doctores y centro de trasplantes.

Pueda que le pegue al Gordo con su siguiente donador y nunca mirar hacia atrás. O el siguiente donador no coincidir con usted pero quizás este dispuesto a participar en el programa de intercambio de riñones. En mi experiencia, yo he tenido pacientes con varios donadores potenciales, los cuales desean participar en el intercambio de riñones, dada la oportunidad y circunstancias. A ti como receptor, esto no solo aumenta sus probabilidades de recibir un riñón y pero quizás lo reciba más rápido.

Así que, recuerda: no te asustes, mantén la esperanza, habla, edúcate a tí mismo, da a conocer tus metas y intenciones, prepárate para un camino largo, persevera, sigue tu régimen medico y una vida saludable, enlístese y busque un donador vivo.

Asi, se obtiene un rinon!

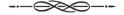

Chapter 14

The Future

In 1975, when I was a renal fellow at UCLA, if someone had told me an unrelated donor with different blood type from a recipient might someday successfully gift a person in need of a kidney transplant with a seemingly mismatched organ, I'd have confidently said, "Don't hold your breath."

Welcome to the 21st century.

For starters, kudos are due to the brilliant research efforts of medical and scientific communities that have given us a far greater understanding of the immune system. New drugs that target certain immune cells, but to some degree, spare others, make renal transplantation more available and successful than ever, extending the life of transplants while decreasing the likelihood of chronic rejection. This alone offers hope to patients awaiting a transplant, along with the success of paired exchanges, blood-type-incompatible transplants and immune-modulating induction therapies.

As noted in the last chapter, Dr. Jochen Reiser, MD, PhD, has developed a device (still in the experimental stage) designed to remove a factor in Focal Segmental Glomerulosclerosis patients, a factor called su-par, which he believes may cause FSG. Though some colleagues have challenged this, he firmly believes that removing su-par can cure FSG.

I'm in close contact with Dr. Reiser, eagerly awaiting his research results.

Meanwhile, researchers led by UC San Francisco bioengineer Shuvo Roy and Vanderbilt University nephrologist William Fissil are developing a surgically implantable artificial kidney that would offer an alternative to dialysis or transplantation.

"We're creating a bio-hybrid device that can mimic a kidney to remove salt and water to keep a patient off dialysis," Dr. Fissil explains. "The implantable artificial kidney, about the size of a soda can, contains microchip filters and living kidney cells, and will be powered by the patient's own heart."

Fine-tuning blood flow to prevent clotting remains a challenge. Dr. Armanda Buck, a biomedical engineer with an interest in fluid mechanics, uses computer models to refine the shape of channels inside the device to achieve the smoothest flow. Then, with the help of 3D printing, a prototype will test how smoothly blood flows through it.

Professor Fissil has a long list of patients eagerly awaiting a chance to participate in trials with the new device. He says, "My patients are absolutely my heroes. They come back again and again, accepting a crushing burden of illness because they want to live. And they're willing to put all of that at risk for the sake of another patient."

Another nascent technology holding great promise for kidney patients is 3D printing, the manufacturing of a three-dimensional object from a computer-driven model. This process is additive, where multiple layers from computer-aided design, are laid down, one after another to create different shapes. Dr. Anthony Atala, is pioneering development of 3D printing of a transplantable kidney with living cells. A bio-printing company is already making human kidney tissue.

Dr. Sharon Presnell, explains, "Our bio-printed human kidney tissue is a significant advance over single-layer cell cultures used today for drug testing. The histologic and functional features of the first prototype are compelling. This means that the cells are functioning with precision and exactly mimic structures in a real kidney."

There is much work to be done before an entire human kidney can be printed and available for transplant. However, I'm confident that someday dialysis units will begin disappearing, thanks to this technology.

Equally important are advances in learning how to prevent kidney disease in the first place. Epigenetics, for example, is a relatively new science that attempts to demonstrate that even our genes, which determine future encounters with certain illnesses, can be modified by lifestyle. The hypothesis is that without changing DNA through a means like gene splicing, one might prevent the expression of a gene through environmental modification.

How? Well, consider diabetes and the relationship between obesity and people genetically predisposed to getting the disease. When fat cells are removed from the equation by eating less and moving and exercising more, the gene may not penetrate, and diabetes may be avoided in some patients. Maintaining a normal **Body Mass Index** (BMI—a person's weight in kilograms divided by the square of height in meters; a high BMI can indicate high body fat) and achieving physical fitness have been shown to reverse pre-diabetes, blocking one of the most common paths to ESRD.

Consider this: A clinical study published in 2018 in the prestigious medical journal *Lancet* followed 306 people in England who had lived with type 2 diabetes for as long as five years. These men and women, all overweight or obese, followed a special diet limiting calories to about 825, by drinking three milk-based shakes—one each for breakfast, lunch, and dinner—for three to five months. The study demonstrated that 46% of the patients became diabetes-free for at least six months, as measured by Hemoglobin A1C levels. They all lost significant weight, attesting to the powerful influence on insulin resistance played by those pernicious adipocytes. These patients have returned to a more normal diet and are being followed closely. This extraordinary study offers hope for any one with type 2 diabetes.

So, I preach again: Doctors should do all they can to convince public-health leaders and state and federal government officials that preventing obesity, diabetes and heart disease—all contributors to ESRD—are attainable goals, Ironically, this common-sense approach is often far more complex than developing stem cells that grow into kidneys, then printed by a 3D printer. Why? Because it starts with education, which, as seen in many areas of public life, is often the toughest challenge and least-funded priority of all.

The future is still brighter and more hopeful than ever for kidney-disease patients. Don't allow fear and suffering to destroy your life. Accept circumstances over which you have no control, and find a bright, compassionate nephrologist who will shepherd you through the sojourn of dialysis and treat it as a means to an end— a renal transplant.

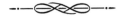

Capítulo 14

El Futuro

En el ano de 1975, cuando cursaba la rotación de nefrología en UCLA, si alguien me hubiera dicho Que algún dia seria posible trasplantar un riñón de una persona con un tipo de sangre diferente a otra persona no compatible inmediatamente diría que eso seria una locura total.

Bueno, los tiempos han cambiado.

Para empezar, es importante destacar los grandes avances científicos que nos han permitido entender mas fondo el sistema inmunológico con nuevos medicamentos que afectan ciertas células inmunes mientras mantiene otras células intactas causando q un trasplante sea tan exitoso como nunca antes , esto a la vez hace q los trasplantes se realicen mas a menudo mientras bajando las probabilidades de ser rechazados por el cuerpo. Esto último ofrece esperanza a pacientes en espera de un trasplante, junto con el éxito del intercambio de pares, tipo-incompatible con sangre de trasplantes y terapias de inducción inmune-modulando ya explicadas anteriormente.

Como se señaló en el capitulo anterior, Dr. Jochen Reiser, MD, PhD, ha desarrollado un dispositivo (aún en fase experimental) diseñado para eliminar un factor en los pacientes de la Glomeruloesclerosis Focal y segmentaria, un factor llamado Su-par, que él cree puede causar FSG. Aunque algunos colegas han cuestionado este método, el cree firmemente que la eliminación de su-par puede curar FSG. Yo estoy en contacto directo con el Dr. Reiser, esperando ansiosamente los resultados de su investigación.

Mientras tanto, los investigadores guiados por el bioingeniero Shuvo Roy de la Universidad de California San Francisco y la Universidad de Vanderbilt como el nefrólogo William Fissil están desarrollando un riñón artificial implantable quirúrgicamente que ofrecería una alternativa a la diálisis o el trasplante.

"Estamos creando un dispositivo de bio-híbrido que puede imitar un riñón para eliminar sal y agua para mantener a un paciente fuera de diálisis", explica el Dr. Fissil. "El riñón artificial implantable, es aproximadamente del tamaño de una lata de soda contiene filtros microscópicos y células biológicas del riñón que serán controladas por el corazón del paciente."

Actualmente, el Profesor Fissil ya tiene una lista larga de pacientes esperando ansiosamente una oportunidad de participar en los ensayos con el nuevo dispositivo. "Mis pacientes son absolutamente mis héroes", dice. «Vuelven repetidas veces, aceptando una carga de la enfermedad porque quieren vivir. Y estan están dispuestos a poner todo eso en riesgo por el bien de otro paciente."

El problema con este dispositivo es el prevenir la coagulación de sangre. Esto si que es un gran desafio. La Dr. Amanda Buck, una ingeniera biomédico con interés en la mecánica de fluidos, utiliza modelos informáticos para perfeccionar la forma de canales dentro del aparato para lograr el flujo de sangre más biológica. Luego, con la ayuda de una impresora 3D, un prototipo, prueba como la sangre fluye por dentro.

Otra tecnología emergente con gran promesa para los pacientes de riñón es la impresora 3D, la fabricación de un objeto tridimensional de un modelo dirigido por ordenador en 3D. Este proceso es aditivo, donde varias capas de diseño asistido por una computadora, se empalman, una tras otra, para crear diferentes formas. El Dr. Anthony Atala, es pionero en el desarrollo de la impresión 3D de un riñón trasplantable con células vivas. Una empresa de bio-impresión 3D ya está haciendo tejido renal humano.

Dr. Sharon Presnell explica: "nuestro tejido de riñón humano bio-impreso es un avance significativo sobre cultivos de células de una sola capa utilizados hoy para las pruebas de drogas. Las características histológicas y funcionales del primer prototipo son prometedoras. Esto significa que las células funcionen con precisión, exactamente imitando las estructuras de un riñón real."

Hay mucho trabajo por delante antes de que un riñón humano pueda ser creado y que sea disponible para el trasplante. Sin embargo, estoy convencido, de que algún día las unidades de diálisis comenzarán a desaparecer, gracias a esta tecnología.

Igualmente importantes son los avances en el aprendizaje de cómo prevenir la enfermedad renal en primer lugar. La Epigenética, por ejemplo, es una ciencia relativamente nueva que intenta demostrar que incluso nuestros genes, que determinan futuro encuentros con ciertas enfermedades, pueden ser modificadas con el simple hecho de cambiar su estilo de vida. La hipótesis es que sin cambiar el ADN , como cortándolo a la mitad , uno puede evitar el desarrollo de muchas enfermedades a través de modificaciones ambientales.

Cómo? bueno, consideren la diabetes y la relación entre la obesidad y en personas genéticamente predispuestas a contraer la enfermedad. Cuando las células de grasa se quitan de este cuadro por comer menos y haciendo mas ejercicio, el gene no se puede desarrollar y la diabetes se pueden evitar en muchos pacientes. Manteniendo un índice de masa corporal normal (BMI) - peso de una persona en kilogramos dividido por el cuadrado de la altura en metros, un BMI alto puede indicar alta grasa) y lograr una condición física han demostrado revertir o prevenir la prediabetes, bloqueando uno de los caminos principales que conducen ala insuficiencia renal.

Por lo tanto, voy a decir esto otra vez. Los médicos deben hacer todo lo posible para convencer a líderes de salud pública y estado y funcionarios del gobierno federal que prevenir la enfermedad de obesidad, diabetes y corazón, todos los colaboradores a ESRD, son metas alcanzables. Irónicamente, este método que tiene mas sentido común a menudo es mucho más complejo que el desarrollo de las células madre que crecen en los riñones, entonces impreso por una impresora 3D. ¿Por qué digo esto? Ya que se inicia con la educación, que, en muchas áreas de la vida pública, es un gran desafío de obtener ya que carece de importancia y recursos financieros. Esa es la realidad.

Sin embargo, puedo decir que el futuro es todavía más brillante, más optimista que nunca, para los pacientes de enfermedad renal. No permitas que el miedo y el sufrimiento destruyan su vida. Usted debe aceptar las circunstancias sobre las cuales no tiene control y buscar un nefrólogo brillante, compasivo que le lo guie por esta travesía de la diálisis y lo trate como un medio hacia un final favorable, un trasplante de riñón.

¿No se conforme con menos, porque nadie mas se va preocupar por uno mas que uno mismo!. Controle su futuro, no dejes que el futuro te controle. Quizás incomodaras a mucha gente inclusive médicos durante todo este proceso. Pero que importa! A nadie le va importa su salud mas que a uno mismo. Pos órale!. Adelante y a echarle ganas. Recuerda esto, tu eres "el amo de tu proprio destino".

Chapter 15

Obesity and Kidney Disease

Obesity has been called the "new cancer," and officially labeled, "The Epidemic of the 21st Century" by the U.S. National Institutes of Health. It is, of course, a primary cause of type 2 diabetes, in turn, the most common cause of End Stage Renal Disease.

Obesity has become such a specter worldwide so fast, it has been compared to the Plague or 'Black Death' that rampaged throughout Europe in the late Middle Ages. Likely, if we don't take steps to reduce it quickly, obesity may well kill far more people. That's how seriously health experts are taking this issue.

I'll offer you some worldwide stats on obesity in a moment, but here are some more unusual facts about the problem that might actually give us a better understanding of how colossal and sometimes confusing the obesity bomb can be, and some reasons behind it. French fries, cookies, cakes, donuts, ice cream, soda and fried foods are at the top of the "kill-you-and-your-children-early" list. Sorry to put it like that, but it's the truth. That's what these "wonderfully-tasting" substances (I can't in good conscience call them "food") do – they kill and not in a nice way.

Now, the disturbing facts: Americans consume 31% more packaged food than fresh food. If you think it's okay to eat "fat foods" in moderation, you've accepted a dangerous and deadly myth. Even moderate weight gain after the age of 20 raises the risk of kidney disease and other major illness.

- At age 50, if you weigh even more than 10 pounds more than you did at age 20 (assuming you had a normal BMI at 20), your risk has grown.

- More than 20 percent of all American meals are eaten in an automobile. Combined with our terrible habits of texting or drinking while driving, it helps explain why 43,000 Americans, and more than one million people worldwide, die each year in traffic accidents.

- Nearly one in four American drivers will have an accident this year, and nearly three million Americans will be injured, according to federal statistics. Turns out, fast food has more than one way to get you.

- For each 10-pound increase in weight gain over your youthful weight, you lower your changes of gaining in a healthy way by 20 percent.

- Extra weight gain is the primary reason people don't age in a healthy way into their 70s.

- At least one out of four people eat fast food every day.

Okay, since my motivation to write this book was to share information about how we can overcome these problems, I've tried to find some silver linings in all these statistics. Maybe one of the better ones is the fact that Americans eat out at fast-food restaurants at a four percent decreased rate than we did in 1995—a small decrease, but better than the opposite.

By the way, I have nothing against the "fast" part of "fast foods" and I don't oppose "drive-through" dinners, but I detest the amount of deadly substances they offer. If they would simply change their menus to offer fresh, healthy food, I'd be a fan. Clearly, we have a long way to go in that regard.

Overall, we're eating out more than ever before, but we dine at what the US Department of Agriculture considers "non-fast-food" restaurants. In the early 1960s, Americans ate at home about 72 percent of the time. Today, that number has shrunk to less than 50 percent. No surprise, then, that the USDA says total sales of fast-food restaurants have risen from $151 billion in 2002, to more than $200 billion in 2016 and may reach $250 billion by 2020.

That's a lot of French fries, a lot of obesity, and a lot of dialysis.

Unfortunately, there's more tough news. Here are some sad and terrifying statistics from the World Health Organization (WHO): Obesity has more than doubled in the past 35 years and is now considered one of the top five causes of death worldwide. More than 40 percent of all adults and more than 41 million children worldwide are overweight or obese. Nearly all of them are candidates for type 2 diabetes. Globally, more people die from being overweight than underweight.

According to the federal Centers for Disease Control, more than one-third of U.S. adults are obese; another third is overweight. That leaves just one-third of Americans close to a weight considered "healthy." More than 80 million adults and 12 million American children are at risk for type 2 diabetes because of being overweight. Never in history have so many Americans knowingly headed for such serious health problems. Obesity-related conditions include heart disease, stroke, type 2 diabetes, hypertension, kidney disease, and certain types of cancer, says the WHO. Others directly linked to obesity include fatty liver and cirrhosis, osteoarthritis, pulmonary disease, and depression.

Most frustrating for medical professionals and anybody who cares about public health? We can avoid nearly all of these future waves of shattering pain and suffering, but we won't make headway curbing this disaster until we recognize its enormity, then focus on solutions. Frankly, our national denial of this massive challenge stuns me, like an earthquake fault that's gashed across our nation, swallowing two-thirds of our citizens, with few paying any attention. Meanwhile, fried, sugary foods and drinks are killing us by the millions.

I'd like to think we're better than this. We can resolve to get healthy again, but we need a massive wake-up call, a realization that not only fulfilling and satisfying, getting in shape and eating good food can be fun. If you stop eating garbage for just a month, you'll likely find you no longer have a taste or longing for it. In fact, even the thought of eating "fat food" will turn your stomach, once you stop consuming it. It's amazing how much better you feel when you choose good food and nutritious drinks for yourself and your children.

The human body is so forgiving, but only to a point. Give it a chance!

The Link Between Obesity and Stress

The link between obesity and stress is well known. Just like many of you, I've reacted to stress at times by wolfing down "comfort foods" like ice cream and bread-and-butter, attempting to assuage pain and discomfort. Bad idea. Fact is, we should eat for nutrition, not comfort. Sometimes, when we're tired, we act on the illusion that eating more will perk us up, but we just get more fatigued as calories accumulate. Eating constantly has little to do with hunger, but is a habitual, mindless reflex to which many of us are drawn when we're bored or stressed. Application of the 21st century term "mindfulness" is appropriate here, because it implies knowledge of the consequences of thoughtless behavior, followed by a thoughtful intention to modify noxious behavior. Knowledge is king, and self- knowledge is the king of kings.

Reasons we've become obese are complex. Some folks are genetically wired to eat excessively, while others are literally trying to fill an internal emptiness that can't be satiated with food alone. The rich aren't immune to the obesity epidemic, however, obesity is common in poorer neighborhoods, where people may not be able to exercise safely, home-cooked meals aren't always available, and they're more likely to eat junk food. These folks tend to be less educated and therefore ignorant of the consequences of their behavior.

In theory, we have free choice. No one forces us to eat unhealthy foods. There are, however, powerful forces at work that interfere with making healthy eating choices. Ignorance tops the list because unless you understand the dangers of eating mindlessly, there's no good reason to change. Why spend more for food that is not as easily available and doesn't taste as good?

Ubiquitous stress plays a mighty role in causing gluttonous eating. Food acts on pleasure centers of the brain, offering temporary respite from the anxiety. Other powerful forces abetting unhealthy eating include food and beverage industries that continue offering relatively inexpensive food, supersized, tasty, and laden with calories derived from sugar and fat. They even hire chemists called "flavorists," to blend salt, fat, and sugar in just the right proportion to entice kids to crave the taste. The caffeine and sugar in soda are by themselves addicting. Excess salt plays a role in generating hypertension in many victims as they gain weight. This variable plays a large role in the genesis of kidney and heart disease.

When family and friends plop in front of the TV watching Sunday football, it's no surprise to see chips dipped in high-calorie dips, pizza, beer, soda, and more. During the many commercials that interrupt the game, we're urged to keep eating and drinking the same class of foods that we're already stuffing into our digestive system. Famous athletes, easily recognized by adults and children alike, bite into mouthwatering double cheeseburgers topped with bacon, muscling them down with sugar-rich soda, implying that if you want to be like us, fit and rich, follow our food habits. Over time, we become programmed to eat this way—in front of the TV, where we sit, sedentary, burning few calories, our bodies steamrolling toward ill health.

Rather than simply blame the food industry as greedy and interested only in their bottom line, we must take responsibility for our choices. I hope that the information to follow will motivate adults to make better eating choices for themselves and their children. A child becomes the victim of a form of child abuse when parents allow that youngster to become obese. Children will always follow their role models, and parents are the greatest influence in most children's lives.

Simply put, we need to gain control, or risk not only a range of horrible diseases, but overwhelming our already-fragile health-care system. Former governor of Arkansas Mike Huckabee, with whom I don't always agree politically, nevertheless made a vitally important statement about his health and America's health. Upset about the state of his own health, he wrote a book about obesity, *"Quit Digging Your Grave with a Knife and a Fork."* He had grown obese and was told he had pre-diabetes but was fortunate enough to get great medical advice from his internist. He lost enough weight to lower his BMI to near-normal and became a marathon runner. His never developed full-blown diabetes. This message needs to resonate with all of us. If we change our approach to life by acquiring knowledge about prevention of chronic illnesses, and act upon it by eliminating addicting, poisonous food and becoming physically active, the incidence of diabetes and diseases associated with neglectful lifestyles will plummet. (An addendum, since I described Huckabee's success in losing weight and avoiding diabetes: He has clearly gained much weight back, demonstrating how difficult it is to maintain normal weight once you've been obese.)

Each of us has the power to shape our destiny, if we have the know-how and the willpower. Certainly, every one of us has the "why" to stay healthy, but frequently lack the "how." If you doubt my words, visit a dialysis unit and speak to patients who didn't have the knowledge to prevent their illnesses. Hopefully, you'll see the common-sense wisdom of prevention and wellness.

Certainly, this message has been delivered to our citizens before. Hundreds of books about stress reduction, dietary modification, and exercise have been written during the past 20 years, and line the self-help shelves of most bookstores. Dr. Oz and others have reached millions on television with this message, but worsening statistics for obesity and diabetes demonstrates the difficulty of managing this problem and making the message stick.

Former First Lady Michelle Obama made teaching families the importance of healthy eating and exercise her primary mission as First Lady. The vegetable garden she created on White House property to emphasize the importance of fresh produce and better food choices for kids has been ripped out by the new administration. Baby steps toward better and healthier lifestyles were symbolically destroyed at a time when the obesity and diabetes epidemic rages. Hopefully, if those of us who care about our families' health make enough noise, we can get the "garden" back, not just symbolically, but by consuming healthy foods throughout America.

So, what do we do? First, realize that you are the only one who really cares about you! The government is not capable nor interested in helping prevent obesity or diabetes. In fact, as I finish this book, the halls of Congress swirl with controversy, investigations of potentially impeachable crimes march forward, and a "sweeping tax-reform bill" threatens a Children's Health Insurance Program that provides medical care to poor childen, many from minority communities most vulnerable to the health epidemics of the 21st century. They will, for certain, be a part of a burgeoning dialysis population soon. Even if you don't like the idea of subsidizing health care for the poor, we will all pay a much higher price for their future health care when they grow chronically ill. This speaks to the notion that we've grown incredibly short-sighted and obsessed with immediate gratification. So, forget the humane part of the formula for kids' health. Consider it, if you wish, an investment in a less costly health care system. Supporting our children now will save health-care dollars later.

When I started the Diabetes Resource Center of Santa Barbara County, we became the first California affiliate of America on the Move (AOM), headquartered at the University of Colorado. They provided pedometers and encouraged walking 10,000 steps a day. Every 2,000 steps equal a mile and burns 100 calories. Burn 3,000 calories, you can lose a pound. Ironically, the sponsor for AOM was Pepsi; no wonder the emphasis was on exercise rather than reduction of sugar and fat!

Pharmaceutical companies want to sell statin drugs to lower cholesterol, discover drugs that reduce appetite, and find better drugs to control blood sugar. "Device" companies have developed gastric bands to surgically reduce appetite and food intake. In some cases, this can be lifesaving. Absurd, however, is the notion that obese children are having a variety of bariatric surgical procedures to lose weight. How about we treat the cause instead of its effect, by preventing childhood obesity in the first place? Pharmaceutical and device companies have no skin in the prevention game. That's up to us—our families, our kids. We and only we can take (or retake) control of our lives.

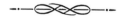

Chapter 16

Prevention and Wellness

Staying well is easier than getting well, the adage goes, and never has it resonated more than today, when, researchers say, 78 percent of chronic diseases affecting 160 million Americans stem from stress, poor diet, lack of exercise, obesity, smoking, and other environmental factors.

Let's start with stress. During more than 40 years of medical practice, I've discerned a link between severe emotional stress and obesity, frequent viral infections, diabetes, cancer, and autoimmune diseases.

Of course, not everyone who endures chronic stress fits into that category. Preparing to write this book, however, I read many histories of other physicians' patients who had kidney transplants, and reviewed my own patients' cases. I found what appeared to be a disproportionate number of patients who had endured severe, prolonged, stress prior to developing an autoimmune disease that caused renal failure. It seemed more than just coincidence. Each had an unusual disease associated with an immune system gone berserk, turning on them, attacking their organs and resulting in the need for lifesaving dialysis.

I discovered, sadly, that many of my patients suffered enormous stress when they were just kids, especially from divorce and/or abusive or neglectful parents. An alarm sounding in my mind lead me to explore what scientists were saying about this connection. After all, the expression "mind-body connection" had been around for many years, but rarely was that term used with young physicians on rounds.

An emerging consensus in a limited segment of the medical community maintains that diseases like lupus, rheumatoid arthritis, psoriatic arthritis, Crohn's disease, multiple sclerosis, and cancer may follow long-term emotional ordeals. In a bit we'll review how the science of psychoneuroimmunology describes possible mechanisms by which stress weakens the immune system and permits the body to turn on itself, causing disease.

Over the past few years, stress has emerged as one of the top five causes of early death, says the World Health Organization. Furthermore, stress and obesity have combined as a terrible twosome. On a molecular level, they both attack most major organs of the body, including the kidneys. In fact, these twin killers often *target* the kidneys, and I often see their destructive path in my own patients. Stress directly causes hypertension and hypertension commonly causes kidney disease, especially in older patients. Stress also promotes obesity, which, in turn, can promote adult-onset diabetes, the most common cause of kidney failure worldwide.

Unlike ancient caveman days, when stress skyrocketed in dangerous situations, then diminished when danger abated, we find ourselves today in world of constant, grinding stress that often doesn't diminish much from week-to-week or year-to-year. The World Health Organization estimates that stress costs American businesses up to three hundred billion dollars a year. The effects of stress on our emotional and physical health, can, of course, devastate adults and children alike. Children suffer far more from stress than many adults realize, and even those who do recognize it are often not exactly sure how to protect their children from it. In an intriguing New York Times Magazine article, Benoit Denizet-Lewis wrote, "More American adolescents than ever suffer from severe anxiety. Parents, therapists, and schools are struggling to figure out why, and whether helping anxious teenagers means protecting them or pushing them to face their fears."

A Stressful Evolution

One of my favorite American writers and philosophers, Henry David Thoreau, witnessed early stages of the modern stress epidemic in the mid-19th century, as the Industrial Revolution accelerated. People worked long hours under intense pressure to succeed in new businesses, many based on emerging, innovative technologies. It began as a strong work ethic, with opportunity to prosper limited only by the need to eat and sleep. Thoreau's advice to "simplify, simplify, simplify," was misunderstood or fell on ears deaf to the birth of the modern-day workaholic. In those days, people were generally ignorant or disdainful of the delicate balance between daily activities humans need to survive and thrive, and the self-inflicted overreach that makes us unhappy and sick. That equation, that delicate balance, remains with us today.

If Thoreau were still alive, he might be appalled, though not surprised, to see that no amount of fame, wealth, or power seems enough for many. An income disparity between the educated and successful and other socioeconomic groups has widened, creating havoc and stress in large swathes of our population. Call it the "stress of the have-nots."

Consider, likewise, highly stressed populations in many communist countries, where an economic gap between workers doesn't exist. Having no say over your destiny, no opportunity for self-advancement or self-governance—call it oppression, if you will—also stresses people out. So, it seems, stress kills capitalists and communists in equal measure. If Thoreau was alive today, I believe he'd agree that freedom—freedom of thought, action, and mobility—is indispensable for healthy people and healthy societies. Combined, they create empowerment, which, with support of family and friends, invites good health. The opposite— chronic and cumulative stress—ultimately destroys rich and poor alike.

The Biology of Stress

Multiple studies have shown that stress has a direct, negative effect on the human heart and on blood pressure. It's becoming increasingly clear, as well, that stress may also attack every other major organ, perhaps whichever one to which our personal DNA has made us the most vulnerable. Kidneys rank high on that list. As major blood-filtering mechanisms of our body, they are highly sensitive to elevated blood pressure and blood sugar. These strain our kidneys, already taxed with a heavy biological workload under normal circumstances. Simply put, high blood pressure and high blood sugar draw a bullseye on our kidneys, waiting only for stress to pull the trigger. The more stress you have, the tighter that finger-grip grows, leaving you ever-closer to catastrophic consequences on your health.

When you arrive home from work, for example, you learn that your spouse has also had a stressful day. Two stressed out people sit down to "decompress" with a glass or two of wine served with cheese and crackers. The kids need attention and the dog barks to get outside, where maybe it hasn't been all day. A report to your company's board of directors is due tomorrow morning. You feel that, in some ways, holding onto your job may depend on that presentation. What's more, a private school in which you have voluntarily enrolled your child begins next month, and it costs the same as if you were sending him to Harvard.

The family that has it all, right? Maybe not. Tonight, sweat trickles, pulses race, and guts tighten as the knock, knock, knock of stress hammers at this couple's door. But, despite the anxiety of pressing circumstances, it didn't show up overnight. The transition from pressure to distress, can take place chronically, subliminally, if a conscious understanding of the role of "balancing" life lies dormant or entirely absent. For example, balance may require spending more time with family (like eating dinner together), living within your financial means, and ditching the purchase of "extras"—trips, toys, and luxury items you can ill-afford and can't take with you after disease drains your spirit, your wallet, your marriage, and your life.

Loss, among so many triggers, commonly feeds the "stress loop." Losing a loved one, a job, a marriage, a sense of self-worth, or any aspect of good health will flood the body with stress hormones—a uniform and universal reaction of the human condition.

As I've said, stress represents an evolved biologic system meant to ready us to overcome immediate danger. The system evolved at least 10,000 years ago during the Stone Age, when small clans of cave-dwellers faced starvation and wild predators. Stress was ubiquitous. The name of the game then was survival. And, to the same degree, but in a different fashion, it still is. Kill or be killed—quite literal for cavemen, applies in equal, more subtle ways to today's world of education, business, employment, and politics. Different environment, same result.

Let's examine the biology of stress—important because with knowledge we can more effectively deflect its deleterious modern-day effects. We can be better partners and parents and remain far healthier. Also, arming your brain will assist you and doctors who know little more than you about stress. So, learn all you can about how it affects you personally and what you can do about it. This can help map a road to prevention and wellness—the cornerstone of a healthy mind, body, and family life, and a sensible mantra for the medical profession.

The moment severe stress strikes, the mind and body respond. It starts in the brain, where a structure called the amygdala senses danger and sends a chemically induced message to the hypothalamus, which acts almost like a command center. It connects with the rest of the body through the autonomic nervous system, which controls respiration, heartbeat, blood pressure, and the dilation and constriction of blood vessels and bronchioles of the lungs. A component of the autonomic nervous system called the sympathetic nervous system initiates the "fight-or-flight" reaction.

Two adrenal glands located just above each kidney respond to the stimulus by secreting cortisol, adrenaline, and noradrenaline. The heart beats faster, the pulse goes up, as does blood pressure. Airways in the lungs dilate to allow maximum oxygen. Epinephrine allows sugar to be released from the liver, while fat is released from storage tissues. Now the individual, in a state of hyper-alertness, is ready to take on challenge. The extent of this reaction is proportional to the immediate threat but results in priming an individual to overcome danger. If the stress doesn't abate, or if it's chronic, the person continues suffering the deleterious influence of cortisol and the autonomic nervous system reaction.

Cortisol released during stress causes insulin resistance, and with ongoing stress it remains at high levels. In addition, during chronic stress, the pancreas is taxed to secrete high levels of the crucial hormone insulin, to prevent very high blood-sugar levels. Essentially, chronic stress creates a state of insulin resistance similar to adult-onset diabetes, as insulin is needed to control blood sugar. If a person has a genetic predisposition for diabetes, he or she is more likely to develop the disease during this period.

Root Causes of Stress

I am not a sociologist or psychologist, but I work daily with patients who suffer negative effects of a stressful life. If I didn't pay close attention to all the pathologies involved with stress, I wouldn't be giving my patients the treatment they really need. Understanding stress and its profound effect on the human body, a focus of mine for some time, remains as important as blood pressure and lab tests for diagnosing and treating disease.

Stress comes from internal and external sources. Let's look first at external stress. Certainly, the modern world brings a crush of digital pressure, ranging from Facebook and Twitter rant to the constant pressure of keeping the machines and electronics that form the fabric of modern life running. Computers, cell phones, all manner of electronic devices, combine to occupy far more brain cells and attention than they deserve. Frankly, I find just keeping my machines working stressful enough, let alone working with them.

Unfortunately, that's merely the tip of the external-stress iceberg. As I noted earlier, we absorb stress from anything that robs us of an ability to have a "say" in our lives. Finances, relationships, loss, and many more sources can inject a deadly river of stress into our bloodstream.

Still, despite the ubiquitous nature of external stress, internal stress can be even deadlier and harder to overcome. Internal stress stems from our own self-image. It's the little gremlin inside us whispering that we are doomed to fail at whatever we do, from jobs to love affairs. We all struggle with some form of it, worse for some than others, where it persists as a terrible, unrelenting generator of pain.

The source of internal stress is complicated and perhaps we are only beginning to learn how messages sent to the brain from the gut play a major role in human health. Still, there's no denying that many of these gremlins emerge in childhood. Dr. Gabor Mate believes that our "wiring," a strong determinate of our behavior, begins early in life and creates a template for all that follows. Neglectful or abusive parents, divorce, and family dysfunction can all play a part. I've heard it from the stories Lupus patients share about their childhoods, when they were subjected to huge amounts of stress they could neither rationalize nor cognitively absorb— typhoons of negativity emanating sour and sordid from an environment where they only expected, only needed, parental love. The same holds true of others who had equally challenging childhoods and adolescent turmoil, then developed other types of autoimmune diseases.

My goal here, however, is not to explain all sources of stress we face. Many great books address that topic, though you need to bring your common sense when you read them (there are plenty of self-proclaimed "gurus" on the subject who advance some far-fetched ideas). If you read carefully, though, you'll get a sense of what your gut and your head tell you, and you'll figure out what information to use and what to disregard.

The cliché that it isn't so much what happens to you in life that matters, but how you deal with it (think Rocky Balboa), rings true here. My Rx for stress? Eliminate as much of it as possible, but more important, learn coping methods. There is no single way to do this. Typically, drugs, alcohol, or any other mind-altering, external substances (or "self-medications") aren't the answer. Better yet: try eating right, yoga, exercise, creating positive relationships, changing your social environment, volunteering, and finding strong purpose and direction in your life. Then maintain all approaches that work for you.

Just remember, unaddressed stress is your worst enemy. Your kidneys, which work so hard for you, plus all your other major organs, depend on it. They deserve your help and you deserve a long, healthy life.

Lethal Links Between Stress, Obesity, and Diabetes

As I mentioned in the previous chapter, obesity has been labeled the "new cancer," and the U.S. National Institutes of Health has called it "The Epidemic of the 21st Century." It's a primary cause of type-2 diabetes, which, says the American Kidney Foundation, is the most common cause of End State Renal Disease.

I've been passionately committed to battling this infirmity and its disastrous consequences for a long time, beginning with what you might call an epiphany I had in 1999, the year I traveled to Leon, Mexico to lecture on strategies for preventing or modifying progressive chronic renal disease. Dr. Allyn and I had worked jointly to develop a state-of-the-art hemodialysis center in Leon, which became one of the first free-standing (non-hospital) units in Mexico. Administered by a team of Mexican doctors, it's still saving lives and promoting kidney transplants.

The lecture preceded a ceremony to celebrate the unit's opening. The future president of Mexico, Governor Vicente Fox, arrived by helicopter to christen the new facility. While preparing to speak, I reviewed relevant medical literature. At the time, most research related to slowing progressive renal failure focused on patients with diabetic kidney disease. Mining the literature, I also discovered an enormous global rise in adult-onset diabetes, matched by a parallel global obesity epidemic.

What shocked me most was that in addition to adults (who, in today's America, average 30 pounds heavier than in the 1960s), obesity among children was rising at an alarming rate, with cases of obese children developing "adult onset diabetes" as early as five years old. This

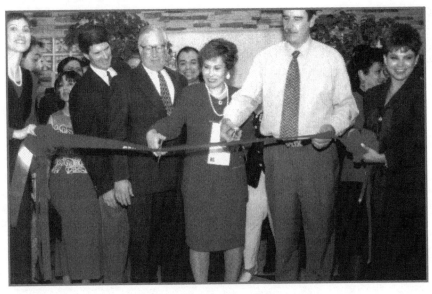

Christening the new facility.

data, a radical departure from health profiles in years past, awakened me to a looming epidemic that would upend the health and wellbeing of children everywhere. My journey to fight this trend began that day, as I visualized young children growing obese through no fault of their own, then becoming diabetics, developing kidney failure, and sitting in dialysis chairs at the Santa Barbara Artificial Kidney Center.
Depressing, to say the least.

The Mexican ceremony was uplifting, meeting Governor Fox a special experience, and giving a speech in Spanish on an important topic exhilarating. But I couldn't extract that searing image of young children growing prematurely diabetic and winding up on dialysis.

I began studying literature related to obesity and the mechanism for its causal role in diabetes. In addition, I reviewed what scholars were saying about childhood and adult-obesity epidemics. What caused this spike in adult obesity during the 1990s and why was it slamming children, too?

To answer the question, let's buckle up for some more science.

Adipocytes, or fat cells, especially ones surrounding the abdomen, aren't just purposeless tissue blobs, sources of social embarrassment. They're complex endocrine organs. Large adipocytes of obese individuals promote inflammation, which many researchers consider the source of nearly all chronic disease. Adipocytes also encourage insulin resistance and thus abet the onset of diabetes.

A hormone called **leptin**, which regulates body fat, also affects weight. Adipocytes release leptin in response to a meal, which signals the brain to make us feel satiated, or "full." Among the overweight, however, leptin's effectiveness declines, so they eat more—a metabolic Catch 22.

Eat more, gain weight, feel hungrier, eat more.

Another fat-cell product, the protein **adiponectin**, promotes normal insulin activity, lowering blood sugar when necessary. Weight-gain diminishes adiponectin levels, encouraging insulin resistance and ultimately type 2 diabetes.

Yet another fat-cell protein, **resistin**, plays a prominent role in causing insulin resistance and, ultimately, diabetes. In fact, in addition to diabetes, resistin fat cells promote cardiovascular disease, hypertension, stroke, high cholesterol, cancer, liver disease, and asthma.

These are some of the metabolic players in obesity and diabetes. Now, let's look at the socioeconomics. Although obesity strikes children of all socioeconomic strata, we find it more among the poor, especially people of color (the two, any sociologist will tell you, often correlate). When experts looked at why this group stood out, it tied directly to omnipresent fast-food chains dominating their neighborhoods.

Looking back at the previous chapter, one of fast-food's strongest draws is that it's, well, fast. It's also inexpensive, tasty, and dense in fat, carbohydrates, and calories. Just a "Big Gulp"-type sugary drink contains up to 500 calories from sugar—33% of what kids need in 24 hours. Moreover, if they consume, say, a Big Mac with their Gulp, that's another 540 calories. Add dessert, a child has exceeded their daily food requirement for healthy growth in one meal. Throw in some greasy, calorie-laden fries, well, you get it.

Back to socioeconomics. Poor people may work two jobs or struggle in single-parent relationships. Often, parents are too tired to fix nutritious meals at night, or healthy foods aren't easily accessible within time constraints of a busy, sometimes deprived, life.

Frequently, poor children live in communities with sprawl, fast traffic, and gangs. It's often unsafe for them to play outside after school. Organized sports are expensive (uniforms and fees), plus they require transport to and from team activities. So, sadly, kids sit at home, glued to TV or the electronic device du jour. Instead of playing sports and games and burning calories outdoors, they spectate.

This is how you become obese. Eat too much, move too little.

With sugar a main component of a sedentary child's diet, a vicious metabolic cycle erupts. Blood-sugar levels rise, the pancreas secretes insulin to lower that level and the child's appetite marches on. The brain, meanwhile, can be fooled to signal hunger instead of satiety when blood sugars first rise and then drop too much, too fast, following a large, sugary meal. Kids wind up eating for comfort, not nutrition.

Despite conflicting data on this subject, it's hard to deny that children who overindulge in high-calorie meals based on sugar and fat become obese, period.

Pre-diabetes, as the name implies, often precedes diabetes. The bad news about pre-diabetes? The patient teeters on the verge of a lifetime spent battling this horrible disease. The good news? Diagnosed early enough, pre-diabetes can be arrested before tail-spinning into full-blown diabetes.

Pre-diabetes is a metabolic state usually seen in obese or overweight people. They often exhibit normal blood sugar levels but elevated insulin levels, signs of a pancreas desperately secreting insulin to maintain normal blood sugar to offset insulin resistance caused by those nasty fat cells.

For the pre-diabetic patient, beating the odds isn't complicated math. By losing 8% body weight, reducing sugar and calorie intake, and exercising, it's possible to prevent onset of type 2 diabetes. Consider this approach two legs of the "health triangle": Exercise, nutrition and rest.

Wouldn't you think knowledge about pre-diabetes would energize a national effort to prevent obesity, the basis of many newly diagnosed cases of adult onset diabetes? Allowing a child to gain 40, 50, 60 pounds of fat cells—each containing myriad protein molecules that lead to diabetes, cancer, heart disease, cirrhosis, arthritis, and emotional distress—seems criminal.

But it's an uphill fight, considering the power of the sugar industry and its lobbyists. The color of money can even lure our finest educational institutions into questionable research with dubious results. In the 1960's, for example, the Sugar Research Foundation sponsored research by Harvard scientists and paid them $50,000 for their trouble. The New England Journal of Medicine published results in 1967. Predictably, the Harvard report minimized other studies implicating sugar as a cause of coronary artery disease and diabetes, blaming fats instead.

You get what you pay for, right? Takeaway lesson: Beware of food-industry-funded studies. Same goes for tobacco, liquor and, okay, I'll say it, guns. Even opioids, the scourge of America's "other" epidemic, were once promoted by pharmaceutical companies as non-addictive.

Home from Mexico in 2000, I was determined to help raise awareness about the menacing epidemic of obesity and diabetes. I started in the place I knew best—Santa Barbara. The city boasts a proud Mexican heritage, with much of its Latino population living in a section called the "eastside corridor." Unfortunately, however, it was a hard place to raise healthy kids. They couldn't walk the neighborhood safely due to relentless traffic and the absence of stop-lights. Gangs were on the rise, with occasional shootings. Milpas Street, the neighborhood's main artery, was (and still is) lined with fast-food restaurants. Liquor stores featuring large candy displays near the cash register, donut shops, and a couple of pizza take-outs dotted the urban landscape.

Adjacent to Franklin School, a neighborhood K-6 elementary facility in the eastside corridor, sits the Franklin Clinic, a provider of family medical care. A large community garden lies across the street. At the north end of Milpas is the Eastside Clinic, also providing medical care.

Memories of my experience as a Peace Corps physician in La Paz, Bolivia, from 1969 to 1971, returned as I considered establishing an obesity/wellness program in the eastside corridor. This is where I would test the hypothesis that childhood obesity could be prevented through education, community buy-in, and cultural awareness. Ultimately, motivating partners like Santa Barbara's mayor, Cottage Health Care's Medical Residency program, UC Santa Barbara, the Superintendent of Schools, local doctors, and the California Medical Association proved critical to the effort.

Make no mistake, however. Though I live and work in Santa Barbara, resources like these can be mobilized to fight childhood obesity anywhere.

In 2000, I also founded the Diabetes Resource Center (DRC) of Santa Barbara County (mentioned in the previous chapter), a non-profit corporation dedicated to reducing the childhood-obesity epidemic in our community. Over time, we raised more than a million dollars from charitable foundations, including the California Endowment, a private health foundation that works to expand access to affordable, quality health care for underserved communities. The DRC worked seamlessly with its partners to help turn the obesity tide in the eastside corridor.

Education about dangers to children and families from childhood obesity was priority number one. We met with community leaders, the Principal of Franklin School, and the mayor. They were all on board.

Predictably, however, there were skeptics.

"You can't change eating or other lifestyle habits stemming from cultural preferences, finances, and deeply rooted habits," they said. Knowing this, and through our relationship with Franklin School and a principal who strongly supported our program, we identified natural community leaders and gave them positions of *Promotoras de Salud* (promoters of health) to help bridge these gaps. They earned small stipends and were thoroughly educated about the dangers of obesity as a cause of diabetes, plus the roles of nutrition and exercise to prevent disease. They understood quickly the enormous danger to their children's wellbeing and zealously pursued their new roles.

Many women became "Tiger Moms," working fiercely to protect their kids' health. They took children on trips to the market, where they learned about processed foods, soda, and reading food labels for calories. Sadly, fresh produce was extremely expensive, making it tough for families to consistently make those healthy choices. Ironically, many dads and other family members worked in the fields, picking the very fruits and vegetables they couldn't afford. Still, the women passed on their acquired knowledge to other community members, and families formed "walking groups" to promote better health.

Franklin School began emphasizing physical education, and specialists came to teach it. The teachers all participated in after-school aerobic classes for their own health and to serve as role models for the students. Campus gardens enriched nutritional and science education.

At the start of the school year all children were weighed, and their heights measured. From those numbers, we calculated each child's BMI. If a BMI is at or above the 85th percentile but below the 95th, the child is overweight. If a child's BMI is greater than 95th percentile, that child is obese.

Baseline data staggered us. Forty-five percent of children entering kindergarten were already overweight or obese. At K-6, 55% of them were overweight or obese—a horrible trend, tragic, in fact, since many of those kids, absent intervention, would likely develop diabetes.

We collected data on the children three times a year. As the program progressed, we saw statistically significant BMI reductions for three straight years. California Governor Arnold Schwarzenegger awarded Franklin School a Gold Medal for its efforts, and Blue Cross, working with the governor, donated a $100,000 state-of-the-art gym, fully equipped with machines geared toward childhood fitness.

The DRC had a small army of volunteers from UC Santa Barbara, Westmont College, and Santa Barbara City College. They helped record BMI's, analyze data, teach sports skills and gardening, and hold fundraisers. It proved an excellent experience, especially for pre-med stu-

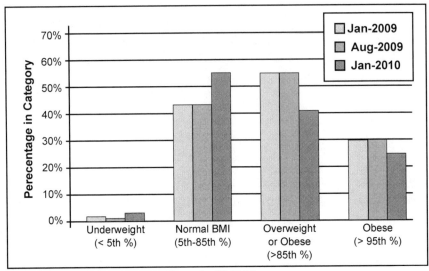

Figure 3: All Children

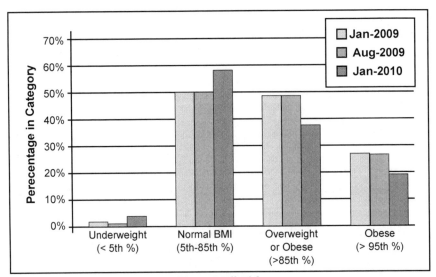

Figure 4: All Girls

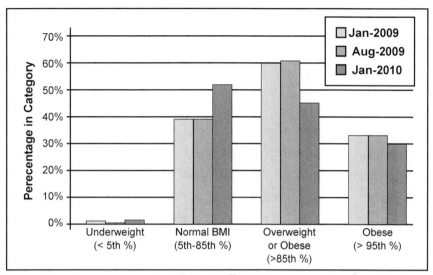

Figure 5: All Boys

dents, to learn about public-health challenges and the scientific roots of obesity. Volunteers earned ongoing teaching opportunities, plus a shot at recommendations to professional schools.

One idea that was never implemented, but that I still believe would have contributed to the Franklin program, was a "wellness prescription." In this model, obese students would visit the Franklin Clinic for medical evaluation, including bloodwork, to establish baseline lipid, blood-sugar and insulin levels, plus a **CRP** (a C-Reactive Protein test detects inflammation, either from an acute event like an infection or from chronic disease that requires further tests to diagnose).

The wellness prescription would also formally involve students in physical activity (including pedometers to count steps and encourage walking) and a nutrition program. *Promotoras de Salud* would help families and children "keep with the program" and encourage parents to follow through with smart food choices at home. Over time, we'd measure and remeasure BMI's, supplementing that data with annual blood work. As BMIs come down, you'd likely see improvement in lipid levels, blood-sugar levels, and inflammatory markers.

When I became ill, however, I dissolved the nonprofit and made Franklin School, already a nonprofit corporation, recipient of all funds directed to the DRC (at this time, however, I'm happy to report that the program is being resurrected). Essentially, this is the Peace Corps model: educate, raise funds, develop programs that work, then let the community take over.

Implementing a program like this isn't easy, especially on a large scale. It will challenge anyone who tries it, especially considering the ceaseless strength of political headwinds. Just like LeBron James slurping Sprite on TV for money, the fast food industry vigorously lobbies to preserve its grip on target communities. Cries of, "Keep the food police out of our lives," and, "We want our freedom" undercut any attempt to reduce junk-food intake and its devastating consequences.

When New York Mayor Michael Bloomberg banned trans-fats from city eateries because they cause cancer, the outcry to keep government out of our lives was deafening. When he proposed reducing the size of sugary sodas (to a "mere" 16 ounces), the soft-drink industry, which, through lobbying and public-relations campaigns had already defeated soda-tax proposals nationwide, challenged the limits in court and won.

Even Senator Bernie Sanders, darling of the progressive left, opposed taxing sugary drinks to make them less available, because, he said, the poor would suffer most. Never mind the fact that kids can drink water. Never mind the steep tax on cigarettes. Nobody says cancer sticks hurt poor people because they're less affordable. Where's the equity, the education, the awareness? Trust me, obesity kills just like cigarettes.

Besides promoting good nutrition, we need exercise, the flip side of the obesity coin. Bluntly stated, America needs to get moving. Taken together, poor eating habits and a sedentary life are a recipe for disaster. Some of my patients say exercise has saved their lives as much as their precious kidney transplants.

"I understand exercise can be challenging," says one patient. "You have to know your body and figure out what works for you. If it's walking, walk. Don't stroll. Walk fast, get your heart-rate up. Bust a bead. Push blood through your entire vascular highway, from large arteries to the smallest capillaries feeding tissue in the farthest reaches of every organ. Exercise isn't just good for your heart. It's good for every part of your body: your eyes, lungs, joints, brain. You name it, exercise helps."

He continues, "If you have joint issues, get in the pool. Lap swimming raises your heart rate and works nearly every muscle in your body. I know, it's cold, it's wet, it may be early in the morning. So, what? You want to live? You want to be healthy? You want to honor your donor? Then get out of bed or off the couch and go after it. If you're not a lap swimmer, try aqua-aerobics. Water, especially the buoyance it provides, allows for non-weight-bearing exercise that you can do well into old-age.

"But whatever you do, however you exercise, do it vigorously at least three hours a week and stick with it. Consider it as essential to your life as brushing your teeth. I know, it's hard, often damn hard. That's why they call it a workout. If it was supposed to be pure fun, they'd call it a fun-out. When it gets difficult, develop a mantra in your head, like "If I can take it, I can make it," or "this pain is just weakness leaving my body."

And always remember: You're stronger than you think.

Once exercise becomes a lifestyle routine, you'll grow addicted to it, in a good way. You'll miss it when you visit grandma for the weekend or when a business trip interferes with your routine. That's your body saying, "I like being healthy; remember to exercise me soon,"

And don't forget the role of exercise to reduce stress. It releases chemicals like endorphins, which make you feel good, "the runner's high," so to speak. And what's better for stress than feeling good?

Other ways to reduce stress, so prevalent into today's frenetic, high-voltage life, include writing, meditating, socializing (don't isolate yourself), and spending time in nature. A walk in the woods, hills, or mountains reminds of us how small we are, matched by how small some of our fears and anxieties may be. It may help you remember not to "sweat the small stuff," especially stuff you can't control that just creates needless stress, which, in turn, feeds disease.

I'm aware, as the saying goes, that "big ships turn slowly," and that some small programs around the nation already focus on reducing obesity. None, however, really incorporate the comprehensive approach necessary to even modestly succeed. So, how do we get there?

I propose a National Health Corps, a Peace-Corps-like program that utilizes the power and intelligence of student volunteers who spend a year in the program before going to college. Consider it a win-win. Volunteers learn public health issues, medicine, cultural sensitivity, and the sociology of poverty, while helping stem the rising tide of childhood obesity.

Let's face it: many young students, even the brightest, head to college not socially mature enough to make their first year meaningful, if they make it at all without returning home overwhelmed. Peer pressure, parties, drinking, and sex, let alone the anxiety of academic expectations and the loneliness of departing home for the great unknown, can wait a year.

That's right, one year, a year spent in a National Health Corps program, a year of (modestly endowed) public service to stimulate maturity, develop a sense of purpose, even gain insight into future careers. Whether the road leads to sociology, anthropology, medicine, or public service, a year of Health-Corps service might beat the value of sitting dazed in a class of 800 being taught by a graduate student, or stumbling confused on the first step of independent life. There's no magic about starting college at 18. Nineteen works just as well, even better, in most cases.

Today's tech world seems obsessed with training the next generation of young entrepreneurs. Emphasis on engineering, business, and computer programming has supplanted commitments to the arts and humanities, essential elements to a full life and a literate, healthy society. Wouldn't it be great if young, exceptional minds lent their intelligence to solving problems that threaten our children and our health care system, even if just for a year?

With Obama's presidency seemingly a distant memory, momentum and enthusiasm about obesity prevention will surely wane (even our current president, the supposed role model and moral compass of our country, proudly displays his fast-food addiction for all to see).

The hot issue of yesterday vaporizes when the vision dims. Like the comfort of a recliner that feels good now but will kill you later, psychic numbness is easier than wrestling bad news, bad policy, and bad outcomes, to the mat. I fear for the families, especially the children, who will just get fatter. And believe me, a chronically unhealthy nation will function and behave poorly.

Now, let's examine links between stress and obesity and how they increase chances for developing diabetes. Our cultural push to "be more," "make more," and "move faster" leads directly to eating quickie "fat foods." Not only unhealthy, these habits undermine core values of the family unit—like eating together around a table. Consider this: The history of words teaches us that food is the fuel of relationships. The word "companion," from the Latin com ("with") and panis ("bread,") reminds us that food—and the brief respite allotted for sharing meals—feeds more than the physical body; it nourishes family and friendship—values that indisputably tighten bonds and decrease stress.

Meanwhile, every 14 minutes another American is added to the kidney transplant list, where more than 100,000 people already mark time, awaiting another chance for a robust life. Most new enrollees in the wait-list "club" come from the half-million patients already on dialysis,

Although stress and overeating clearly damage our health, human factors behind why and how we become obese aren't always simple. Before I address those factors, however, I offer this: with deconditioning techniques, you can utilize the brain's "plasticity," the ability to change in ways not completely understood, to resist temptation and make better choices. The result is self-control and movement toward a healthier lifestyle. Yoga and meditation that focus on breathing, for example, have changed my life. The results have been magical, empowering a resistance to self-destructive behavior. This, in turn, relates to the notion that exercise in general, and the deep breathing it induces, help clear and focus the mind to a point where enhanced wellness and clarity of thought beget smarter lifestyle choices. Think of it like the reverse of stress causing overeating and disease. Relieving stress through exercise and deep breathing clears the mind to make sensible choices, which make you feel better and eager to do it again.

People need knowledge, not only of the grave, self-inflicted consequences of obesity, but how to prevent it in the first place: techniques such as meditation and yoga are good examples. For many people, lifestyle changes remain a daunting task. It's not uncommon, for example, for people to become inflexible and unwilling to try something foreign like yoga, hiking, swimming, weights, walking in nature—anything that stimulates the brain to hit the "reset" button, not the "comfort" button that leads to self-destruction. They often paddle against the tide just to maintain a semblance of order in their lives, so suggesting something that seems so "far out" as yoga can be quickly rejected. When I suggested that children incorporate breathing techniques and yoga during the school day because of its myriad benefits, some parents protested that they did not want a new "religion" introduced to the children. A new religion? Are you kidding me?

I hear Thoreau crying out, "Educate, educate, educate!"

Application of the 21st century term "mindfulness" seems quite appropriate here because it implies knowledge of the consequences of thoughtless actions, compared to a mindful intention to modify noxious behavior. Knowledge, especially self-knowledge, remains king.

Besides an abundance of stress and lack of education, reasons for obesity can be complex. Some folks are genetically programmed to eat excessively while others are literally trying to fill an emptiness that can't be satiated with food alone, but they try nonetheless. The rich are not immune, though obesity is more common in poorer neighborhoods where people may not be able to exercise (due to safety, location, or time constraints) and are more likely to eat junk food. The U.C.L.A. School of Public Health reports that obesity correlates directly with poverty.

One recent study linking poverty to obesity suggests that poor parents allow their kids to eat fatty, sugary foods because these items are more affordable than healthy foods and provide a way for parents to say "yes" in households where "no" is the norm for so many items they can't afford.

Making matters worse, the food and beverage industries prey on the poor, a notion we touched on in the last chapter, but warrants brief re-visitation here. Remember the "flavorists"? Well, the sugar and fat industry giants aren't shy to hire Madison Avenue types to push this lies, and even sponsor now-debunked studies suggesting "their" products don't cause obesity (companies pushing fat blame sugar and vice versa), just like pharmaceutical companies pushing opioids have claimed their drugs aren't addictive. (Frankly, these kind of corporate ruses, undertaken to make huge profit at the expense of public health, stress me out. That's when I need some yoga.)

But absent yoga right now, I'll vent instead: My wife and I recently visited Dodger Stadium for a baseball game. We were horrified to see the oversized bodies of parents, along with their overweight children looking like miniatures of their parents, trudging along with a sugary drink or a huge cup of beer. It seemed like 40% of the adults and children were overweight (the stadium even boasts an "all you can eat" section—and patrons do just that). Sadly, many of the families were Latino, at even greater risk for obesity-related diabetes. In fact, Asian Americans, African Americans, Native Americans, and Latinos are all genetically prone to diabetes. Obesity makes it a near-certainty.

Forgive the preaching, but my convictions on this topic are immutable. Each of us can shape our destiny if we have the knowhow. Certainly, everybody has the "why" to stay healthy, but frequently lack the "how." If you doubt the reality and gravity of my words, visit a dialysis unit, look around, speak to patients who didn't have the knowledge to prevent their illnesses. Hopefully, you'll see the common-sense wisdom of prevention and wellness. Embrace it!

So, what's the likely future for Sunday couch potatoes who crave weekend sporting events as relief from a stressful week, or hit the "all you can eat" section at the ballpark? The same stress that resulted in a high-cortisol state frequently directs many of us to eat mindlessly, at any time of day or night, hungry or not, especially during amped-up, high-adrenaline times like when we watch sports. The die is now cast, seeds sown, for catastrophic illnesses if this process advances unabated.

Fast-forward a decade. Mr. Football is overweight, approaching obesity. He has been experiencing anxiety and low energy. He has just been diagnosed with diabetes, hypertension, and high cholesterol. Not only is the level of cortisol in his blood chronically elevated, reflecting ongoing stress and interfering with the ability of his natural insulin to maintain normal blood sugar, his burgeoning fat cells now act like pernicious endocrine organs, delivering multiple hormones and bioactive proteins into the blood that not only create more insulin resistance, but promote inflammation, hypertension, high cholesterol, even cancer.

This poor soul is now a walking time bomb that will surely detonate, leaving him with serious illness or worse. I've seen this tragic, though preventable, series of events land myriad patients on dialysis.

Autoimmune Disease, Stress, and Cancer

The immune system's job is to protect us from disease by neutralizing foreign antigens like viruses, bacteria, even cancer cells. Chronic and severe stress in vulnerable individuals may reverse its protective role, causing the immune system to attack the body it was designed to protect. Disorders that follow are a spectrum of bizarre maladies called autoimmune diseases.

Is there evidence that stress can modulate the immune system, resulting in autoimmune disease? What, precisely, is the role of relentless stress as a causal factor and what is the pathophysiology by which it accomplishes it?

In 1964, a field of inquiry rooted in the suspected relationship between the brain, the nervous system, and immune response, emerged—a concept dating back to the Greek philosopher Aristotle. Dr. Robert Ader, Director of the Division of Behavioral and Psychosocial Medicine at the University of Rochester, developed the new field of psychoneuroimmunology, devoted to understanding interactions between the immune system, central nervous system, and endocrine system, plus the relationship between physical wellbeing, the brain, and emotions.

I'll refrain from detailing the very complex physiology of our immune system, but instead summarize what we know about how stress can interfere with its actions and render it self-destructive. Chronic stress causes a generalized immunosuppressive effect that reduces the body's ability to deliver an effective immune reaction. A high level of cortisol, which is very much like taking the corticosteroid prednisone, weakens immunocompetence, or the immune system's ability to make appropriate antibodies to a foreign protein invading the body, like a viral or bacterial infection. In fact, prednisone is a drug often used in combination with others to prevent rejection of a transplanted kidney because of its immunosuppressive properties.

The **thymus** gland is an organ located just behind the sternum, or breastbone. Experiments with highly stressed rats show that their thymus involutes, or shrinks, when the animal is exposed to severe stress. What makes this a critical observation? The thymus gland is responsible for the production of T cells, those specialized cells that allow us to fight infections. When the system goes awry from stress, it can result in antibodies attacking the host's own tissues. This defines autoimmune disease.

One disease, rheumatoid arthritis, is associated with an immune marker in the blood called a rheumatoid factor. Not all people who test positive for the rheumatoid factor develop rheumatoid arthritis. It has been suggested, however, that this disease, in which the body makes an-tibodies to its own tissue, is, in some people, induced by chronic stress. I believe it, and I've got company. Dr. William Osler, the author of the first textbook of medicine in 1892, studied many patients with clinical symptoms of rheumatoid arthritis and concluded that more than likely stress played a major role in activating this disease.

Systemic lupus, a much different illness than rheumatoid arthritis, may also be initiated by chronic stress but other variables must be pres-ent for this to occur, otherwise we would have an epidemic of autoim-mune disease. It has been proposed that the specific nature of an indi-vidual's genome and exposure to a specific environmental antigen such as a particular viral infection, in the presence of the crippling stress like the kind Sarah endured, might trigger the onset of Lupus or other immunologic disease such as the pulmonary-renal syndrome that de-stroyed Clare's kidney function. Under stress, certain viral infections may grow more virulent and more likely to trigger violent diseases.

When reading the New England Journal of Medicine CPC (Clinical Pathologic Conference) about the case of individuals presenting with au-toimmune disease, I recall their histories leading to onset of the illness. A couple months prior to the autoimmune disease's manifestation, all of the patients suffered from a "flu-like illness." The set of symptoms de-scribed as a flu syndrome may have been caused by a viral infection that stimulated the immune system to behave aberrantly and wreak chaos in the form of auto immune disease.

This mirrors exactly the clinical progression I've seen in many pa-tients who lived under chronic stress and were exposed to a viral or flu-like illness prior to the onset of systemic lupus. Is this indisputable proof of cause and effect? Probably not, but common sense suggests that recognizing stress and utilizing stress-reduction techniques may be valuable to limiting possible resultant illnesses. Just as we should feed our children healthy, fresh food, we should explore methods to recognize early childhood stress and equip kids and their parents with tools to prevent or preempt diseases like systemic lupus and diabetes.

Parents need to be aware that even mild stress in children may manifest in subtle signs and symptoms. In a 3rd grader feeling stress because of difficulty connecting socially with other children, the only warning to parents may be a mild belly ache, bed wetting, or not wanting to go to school. However, if financial or marital difficulty loom over the child, assume he or she will feel severe stress. The best approach to this is simply talking to, consoling, and carefully observing your child for changes in mood and behavior. If the disruptive situation persists, speak to the child's pediatrician and seek emotional support early.

Educating parents to recognize significant stress within the family unit, while also understanding its danger if left unabated, is critical. The application of stress reduction techniques, may avert serious consequences. Early counseling, effective use of breathing techniques, meditation, yoga, walking, or just "talking it through" are all effective. Prevention and wellness should be a mantra. It best begins in childhood, but the entire family needs it and benefits from it.

Stress, Obesity, and Politics

I'm manifestly frustrated about the state of our nation's health, which isn't likely to improve anytime soon. The stress, diabetes, obesity, heart disease, and kidney-failure epidemics will continue to cripple more Americans, harm families, and destroy our already-fragile health care system, which, sadly, our dysfunctional government is incapable of fixing. Powerful insurance-company lobbyists swoop down on lawmakers, paralyzing or strangling any reforms rooted in moral rectitude. Partisan politics, pushed by lawmakers more interested in reelection than public health, prevent Congress from crafting a health care system that benefits all Americans.

Meanwhile, our population of elderly and chronically ill patients, many of whom have diabetes, heart disease, and renal failure, continues to grow. This places a larger burden on doctors, already under siege from a burgeoning patient population and strangling red tape. How sad it is when your physician sits in front of you taking a medical history with his face staring down at a laptop computer, hastily typing in key words needed for a required report just be compensated for the care. How can he or she find time to discuss the role of exercise, nutrition, and stress-reduction for patients most in need, with that time squeezed by mundane actions that are required just to ensure payment? The patient feels a lack of caring and connection. Both doctor and patient feel the stress generated by a perverse system and its misplaced values. In the end, the patient suffers the consequences.

It's no surprise, meanwhile, that many physicians are opting for a cash-only, boutique-style "concierge" practice, in which they do not accept insurance, make themselves available, and try to practice "old-style medicine" based on trust and intimacy, never having to worry about billing and other annoyances that diminish the doctor-patient relationship. The result is high-quality care that all patients deserve. The downside? It only pays for your doctor and his/her services. You still must pay for lab tests, treatments, hospital visits, and more. So, the cash-strapped need not apply, and the disparity in health benefits between wealthy and poor only grows wider.

To young adults and young parents: First, accept the notion that stress will always be present—not a scare tactic, a fact of life. Plan strategies in advance to deflect whatever comes your way. Stay in tune with your body, which will speak to you if you abuse it. Learn to trust what your body says and avoid obvious activities that cause malaise. Kids: Early recognition of stress create opportunities to talk to your parents and friends. For parents, consider a psychologist who can deliver important tools that allow couples to work together as problem solvers, for you *and* your kids.

Teaching children, early on, to perceive subtle stress and develop a simple stress-reduction strategy to address it, can equip them with tools that they can use over a lifetime. Dr. James Doty, professor of Neurosurgery at Stanford University and Director of the Center for Compassion and Altruism Research, wrote a book called Into the Magic Shop. He was very poor growing up and came from a dysfunctional home. How did he overcome this suffocating stress to reach such success? A powerful mentor taught him the technique of meditation and intelligent breathing when he was 12 years old. Before spending an entire summer under her mentorship, he was failing in school with no interest in attending college. I strongly recommend this book to anybody who wants to learn how the mind can be reprogramed to effectively handle even the most noxious stress—especially parents who struggle to learn their role in their kids' challenges and want to help reduce stress that may be choking their whole family. Likewise, the brain's plasticity allows reprogramming to eat healthy foods, exercise, and avoid self-destructive behavior.

I attended a Hindu service in the home of one of my nephrology partners. At the end of the ritual, the pundit spoke to the parents and children, aiming to leave them with pragmatic lessons from the ceremony. He suggested parents should make children aware of their breathing, a rhythmic constant, a source of life, as a potentially powerful tool to combat stress. Parents who are aware and sensitive to the mood of their kids can teach a child to sit for 3-5 minutes in the presence of obvious stress, to simply focus on the in-and-out of breathing. I suggest using this technique not only for stress relief, but as part of a daily routine.

Pranayama is a Sanskrit word that describes breathing. *Prana* means breath and *yama* means life. Focusing on incorporating ancient techniques introduced by the Yogis may lower blood pressure, slow the heart rate, reduce respiratory rate, and help calm the nerves. Even when all is calm, a few moments of stillness, focusing on breathing, away from distraction, provides immediate benefit and a tool for handling all that life throws at you.

Yoga has been a blessing for me, both as a stress reducer and to remain strong, flexible, and relaxed. Two months after my lung surgery, I was back in the yoga studio where I regained strength, self-confidence, and awareness of how I could improve my breathing and utilize it to relax. I strongly suggest young families incorporate yoga, martial arts, meditation and other Eastern disciplines as lifelong strategies to reduce stress and remain healthy. Swimming, tennis, and running are excellent too—they defy shallow breathing, forcing the lungs to expand, the diaphragm to expand and the blood to flow, all ways to nourish a stressed soul.

A recent article in the Harvard Health Blog described studies on yoga's effects on stress. One study, in the journal Oxidative Medicine and Cellular Longevity, found that 12 weeks of yoga slowed cellular aging. The program consisted of 90 minutes of yoga, five days a week for 12 weeks, and included physical postures, breathing, and meditation. Researchers found lower levels of inflammation markers (the inter-cellular building blocks of disease), as well as lower levels of the stress hormone cortisol. Another biomarker found in the brain is Derived Neurotrophic Factor, or BDNF, a naturally occurring protein in the body that regulates neuroplasticity and promotes brain development. The study found higher levels of BDNF after the yoga program, suggesting yoga may protect the brain as well.

Throughout this book I've summoned fifty years of medical experience to advance the notion that unabated stress alters our body functions and makes development of life- threatening, chronic disease more likely. I've drawn attention to the science of psychoneuroimmunology where evidence continues accumulating to support my observations.

To additionally support my observations let me share some important and potentially very hopeful news for those who have kidney disease and need a transplant, and for those already living with a successful transplant.

Although I cannot divulge many details yet, one of my kidney-transplant patients is participating in a clinical trial, the purpose of the which is to test protocols for preventing chronic rejection, which may be caused by host-specific antibodies and may lead to kidney dysfunction or loss several years post-transplant. The test involves an injectable drug that works by blocking a receptor for a cytokine called interleukin 6. Interleukin 6 is made by immune cells and causes inflammation. In a transplanted kidney, it can lead to loss of kidney function.

Additionally, here's some more scientific evidence of how the mind, through meditation, can reduce inflammation by reducing levels of interleukin 6. In March 2018, a study published in "Biologic Psychiatry", reported on two groups. Both had blood work for inflammatory markers including Interleukin 6. Four months later, the group that practiced meditation had significantly lower levels of all inflammatory markers including interleukin 6. I have asked my patient to practice mediation as an adjunct to his experimental interleukin 6 inhibitor. This important study should encourage all of us to fend off stress with "mindfulness."

Now, let's circle back once more—I promise, just once more—to food and exercise. Learn to shop the periphery of supermarket aisles, where fresher produce and healthier foods hide (crazy, how you must navigate through processed food to the healthy stuff). Never bring soda into the house. Teach your kids that berries, melon, yogurt, and other fruits are dessert. Drink water, which has an appetite-killing effect. Avoid fruit juice—it's very caloric and sugar-rich. Eat an orange instead of drinking orange juice or at least dilute the fruit juice with water. An apple before a big meal dampens the appetite effectively and has a low glycemic index. Avoid processed foods if possible, but of course be flexible around birthday parties and other celebrations. Eat slowly. Enjoy the resultant family conversation—so rare in today's fast-paced life. Eating slowly allows food to absorb and signals the brain that you're satisfied. Be great role models for children who follow your lead.

Again, exercise in any form is crucial for a healthy body and mind. Not only are calories used during movement, but hormones spill from the brain, reducing stress and making you feel well. Effective time management allows for exercise every day. In fact, if you take even 30 minutes to exercise, you'll be far more efficient at whatever task to which you return. When I played basketball on weekends as a medical student, I felt better and was able to accomplish much more when I returned to the library afterward. In retrospect, I'd have fared even better if I had played more often.

Families: Make a covenant with your doctors and pediatricians to work together to encourage a healthy lifestyle aimed at preventing unnecessary, even life-threatening illnesses. We tend to only see our doctor when we are sick, rendering ever-so-easy a tendency to stray from the discipline required to maintain normal body weight, good nutrition, healthy eating habits, and exercise, and to learn to recognize the earliest effects of stress. At the very least, visit your doctor annually— for checkups, baseline comparisons, and ongoing assessment of where you've been, where you are, and where you need to be. Making this a priority will reap lifelong benefits.

Honestly, I wish I had the information I'm sharing with you when I was a child or young adult. I was clueless about the power of epigenetics or changing an unhealthy lifestyle, modifying diet, modifying the penetrance of "bad" genes. The best example of this is worth repeating because it should leave all of you with hope. If you are overweight and have a family history of diabetes you do not have to become a full-blown diabetic. If you are still in the pre-diabetes phase and lose 8% of your body weight, begin exercising, continue this healthy behavior, and apply stress-reduction techniques, you can avoid a life sentence, or, worse yet, a death sentence.

It's never too late to learn and grow. I've adhered to the healthiest lifestyle possible since I absorbed and embraced this information. Despite my serious medical history, I've never felt better. I'm off all meds that modulate my immune system, eat in moderation, eat foods that promote health, keep my BMI in the normal range and practice yoga, lift weights, hike, swim, and play tennis. Pranayama is a go-to when stress comes knocking. The severe diverticulitis, which likely lead to central serous retinopathy and psoriatic arthritis, necessitated the use of the powerful immunosuppressive drugs, Embrel and Humira, to "cool" my very inflamed joints, which are in complete remission now.

But my story doesn't have to be your story. Don't wait for a medical "wake-up call." Act now and that alarm bell will never ring.

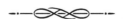

Capítulo 16

Prevención y Bienestar

Como dice el refrán, estar bien es más fácil que mantenerse bien, y esto nunca ha resonado tanto como hoy, por eso es que los investigadores dicen, que 78% de las enfermedades crónicas que afectan a 160 millones de estadounidenses provienen de una mala dieta, falta de ejercicio, fumar, estrés y otros factores ambientales.

Déjenme hablar del estrés. Volviendo a los capítulos anteriores, vemos un patrón, una relación entre estrés y enfermedad. ¿Me pregunto, puede el estrés modular el sistema inmune?

Con más de 40 años de práctica, he discernido un vínculo entre el estrés emocional severo y enfermedades autoinmunes como la de Claire. Los registros de muchos pacientes que recibieron trasplantes de riñón parecen confirmarlo. Todos tenían un común denominador. Cada uno tenía una enfermedad extraña asociada a un desorden del sistema inmunológico que se descontrolaba, girando en el individuo y atacando a sus órganos. No me sorprendió al descubrir que muchos de mis pacientes eran jóvenes, cuyos padres se divorciaron cuando eran chicos.

Un consenso en la comunidad médica, aunque no todavía empíricamente comprobado, indica que enfermedades como la artritis reumatoide, artritis psoriásica, lupus, esclerosis múltiple incluso pueden conducir a muchos trastornos emocionales. Además, una infección viral puede contribuir a la mezcla, atacando a un paciente estresado antes del inicio de la enfermedad autoinmune.

Me pregunto ¿Por qué un evento social como el divorcio pudo haber contribuido a la enfermedad de Claire? Porque se presenta como un precursor que a menudo seria pura coincidencia. Sarah y Claire son dos ejemplos clásicos.

Tengo varios pacientes con historias como la de ellos, todas mujeres que tenían nefritis lúpica grave, insuficiencia renal y trasplantes exitosos. Pero también hubo una excepción: un hombre, lo cual es menos común. Aún así, el común denominador común sigue siendo el mismo, él, también, paso por un divorcio antes de su enfermedad renal.

He hablado con colegas que tratan a los pacientes con lupus y otros trastornos del sistema inmunológico, principalmente reumatólogos y nefrólogos. Les pedí revisar historias de pacientes en los últimos 30 años para ver si compartían la impresión de que el estrés es un componente o un precursor de enfermedades autoinmune.

La respuesta, aunque no unánime, fue «Sí». ¿Cual es mi punto de vista personal? Es clarísimo que el estrés promueve al desarrollo de enfermedades.

Mientras tanto, la insuficiencia renal causada por diabetes se encuentra en medio de esta enojosa tendencia de "enfermedad de estilo de vida" que amenaza con abrumar a nuestro sistema de salud y presupuesto financiero de salud. De hecho, alrededor del 30 por ciento de los pacientes con diabetes tipo 1 (juvenil) y 10-40% de los pacientes con diabetes tipo 2 (comienzo adulto) sufrirían insuficiencia renal debido a esta enfermedad renal la cual es completamente prevenible. Y como nuestras familias, disminuyendo las filas de los que "temporalmente están sanos," la devastadora diabetes invita a otras complicaciones como ceguera, enfermedades del corazón, enfermedad vascular periférica y amputaciones de extremidades.

La diabetes ha alcanzado una proporción epidémica difícil de frenar. Puesto que es la principal causa de insuficiencia renal, incurables una vez que se apodera de la persona, debemos *cortar debajo de las rodil-*

las antes de que continúe arruinando nuestros cuerpos y vidas.

En una nota moral, los padres deben aprender la función que tiene la nutrición y el ejercicio para prevenir terribles enfermedades como la obesidad y la diabetes, por no hacerlo seguirá matando nuestros mas seres queridos. Es una propuesta simple: Cuida tus hijos y mantenlos saludables. Aprende a hacerlo en caso de que no sepas cómo. Esto es parte de ser buenos padres.

¿En comparación, si un padre le da a un niño bebidas alcohólicas temprano en su infancia, eso es maltrato infantil, verdad? ¿Así, si un padre pone un frasco destinado a leche pero lleno de Coca Cola en la boca de un bebé, no es lo mismo? Al hacer esto, el niño ingiere un cóctel de cafeína y azúcar masivo, invitando a la adicción antes de que incluso pueda decir sus primeras palabras. Con mucha frecuencia he visto esto, especialmente en las comunidades pobres. Los padres que no sueñan con golpear a un niño pequeño, sin saberlo los golpean con una nutrición horrible, la cual es el primer paso hacia las enfermedades crónicas e incurables.

Diabetes y sus consecuencias son a menudo prevenibles o controlables, pero, sé que no hay otra manera de decirlo — políticos, congresistas y las mega-corporaciones nos bombardean con alimentos que matan, bloquean el camino a una reforma de salud sanitaria, especialmente la educación sobre los beneficios de la buena nutrición y consecuencias de la mala nutrición.

Estas companias están forradas de dinero. Companias de sodas, por ejemplo, han invertido $ 67 millones en campañas anti-soda-impuestos a nivel estatal y local desde el año 2000. Y miren que ellos patrocinan. LeBron James empuja Sprite. Otros pesos pesados del deporte como Venus y Serena Williams, Eli y Peyton Manning, Apolo Ohno y Shaquille O'Neal publicitación toda clase de comida basura, incluyendo galletas Triple doble Oreos.

Y hay otras empresas de alimentos azucarados no sólo son ricas, pero avariciosas y audaces. Cuando los niños ven este personaje todo sudado LeBron James tomando un Sprite, invitan a que los niños sean como él. Francamente, esto es un envenenamiento de nuestra juventud a través del personajes iconos de deportes lo cual nada mas y menos siembran una trampa para que nuestros chicos caigan y consumas sus productos. Esto es algo manipulativo e incluso inmoral.

En México, donde enfermedades relacionadas con la obesidad mata más gente que el crimen, los legisladores impusieron impuestos a refrescos azucarados en 2014. Ahora, funcionarios del gobierno detrás de esta medidas , además de ser sin fines de lucro promoviendo la buena nutrición, se encuentran acorralados por los opositores de la medida, que usan programas de Spyware para infiltrarse en los teléfonos y otros medios de comunicación. ¿Principales sospechosos? Gigantes de soda que se opusieron a los impuestos, entonces intentaron conseguirlo por la mitad y ahora se oponen a un esfuerzo nacional que se doble el impuesto.

Hoy, la mayoría de los pacientes nuevos que empiezan diálisis en el centro de riñón Artificial de Santa Barbara es a consecuencia de diabetes tipo 2 con insuficiencia renal. Pero hay esperanza. Con 13 millones de niños corren el riesgo de resultados similares, cambiando sus conductas de dieta y ejercicio puede ayudar a evitar enfermedades del riñón.

Con esto en mente, déjenme platicarles una experiencia particular que me intereso con mucha pasion.. En 1999 viajé a León, Gto a dar una

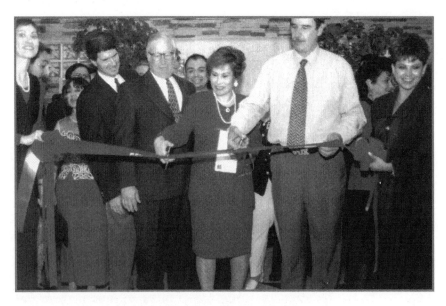

Bautizo de la nueva instalación.

conferencia sobre estrategias para prevenir o modificar la enfermedad renal crónicas. Dr. Allyn y yo trabajamos conjuntamente para desarrollar un centro de hemodiálisis con la ultima tecnología en Leon, que se convirtió en una de las primeras unidades de independiente (no hospital) en México. Ahora en la actualidad es administrado por un equipo de médicos mexicanos, que salvan vidas y promueven los trasplantes de riñón.

La Conferencia fue seguida por a una ceremonia para celebrar la apertura de la clinica. El futuro Presidente de México, que en aquel entonces era el gobernador Vicente Fox, llegó en helicóptero a inaugurar la nueva clínica. Mientras se preparaba para hablar, revisé la literatura médica pertinente. Al tiempo, mayoría de las investigaciones relacionadas con retraso la falta renal progresiva se centró en pacientes con nefropatía diabética. En ese entonces descubrió un enorme aumento global de la diabetes en adultos y una epidemia de obesidad mundial paralela.

Lo que me sorprendió más era además la cantidad de adultos (que, en Estados Unidos de hoy, media 30 libras más pesados que en la década de 1960), la obesidad entre los niños fue aumentando de forma alarmante porcentaje de casos de niños obesos en desarrollo "diabetes de inicio adulto" tan pronto como cinco años de edad. Estos datos, una salida radical de los perfiles de salud en años anteriores, me despertaron una epidemia inminente que le voltea la salud y el bienestar de los niños en todas partes.

Tipo 1 o diabetes juvenil, incluye 5% de la diabetes todos. Ha asociado con un desorden inmune que ataca el páncreas de un niño, destruyendo su capacidad de secretar insulina. El único tratamiento es el reemplazo de la insulina inyectada a diario. Tipo 2, diabetes en adultos, representa el 95% de los casos de diabetes. Se relaciona con un trastorno metabólico complejo que se traduce en grados variables de resistencia a la insulina. Los niveles de insulina comienzan normal, pero el páncreas debe trabajar más duro para el control de azúcar en la sangre secretando más para superar la resistencia de aumento provocada por todo lo de la infección al estrés o usted lo adivinó, obesidad.

Y la obesidad ¿qué hacer con la enfermedad de diabetes y riñón?

En primer lugar, existe una relación linear entre la obesidad y la diabetes de inicio adulto, especialmente para alguien genéticamente predispuestas a desarrollar la enfermedad. Tomado por separado, la obesidad o la diabetes pueden alterar la función renal normal. Combinadas y descontroladas ciertamente conducen a causar enfermedades renales.

En México, una epifanía me llamó la atención que alteró el curso de mi práctica. De repente, había visualizado niños creciendo obesos sin culpa, entonces convertirse en diabéticos, desarrollo de insuficiencia renal y en sentarse en sillas de hemodialisis en el centro de riñón Artificial de Santa Barbara. Esto fue algo muy deprimidor.

La ceremonia fue alentadora, conocer al gobernador Fox fue una experiencia especial y dando un discurso en Español sobre un tema importante y estimulante. Pero yo no pude extraer esa imagen ardiente de niños crecer prematuramente con diabetes y terminar en diálisis a muy temprana edad.

Comencé a estudiar la literatura relacionada con la obesidad y el mecanismo para su papel causal en la diabetes. Además, revisé lo que decían los estudios en ese entonces sobre la infancia y las epidemias de obesidad en los adultos. ¿Qué causó este incremento en obesidad adulta durante la década de 1990 y por qué esta afectando a jóvenes también?

Para responder a esa pregunta, vamos los invito a aprender un poco más sobre la ciencia.

Adipocitos o células grasas, especialmente las que rodean el abdomen, no sólo sin propósito tejido blobs, fuentes de la vergüenza social. Son órganos endocrinos complejos. Adipocitos grandes de individuos obesos promoción la inflamación, que muchos investigadores consideran la fuente de casi todas las enfermedades crónicas. Adipocitos también fomentar la resistencia a la insulina y así instigar a la aparición de la diabetes.

Una hormona llamada **leptina**, que regula la grasa del cuerpo, también afecta al peso. Adipocitos liberan leptina en respuesta a una comida, que señala al cerebro que nos hacen sentir saciados, o "lleno". Entre la persona obesa, sin embargo, la eficacia de la leptina disminuye, por lo que comen más — un metabolismo sin control que hace que la persona coma mas, suba de peso, con mas hambre y comer mas.

Otro producto de la célula grasa, la proteína **adiponectina**, promueve la actividad normal de la insulina, la cual, reduce la azúcar en la sangre cuando sea necesario. Desafortunadamente, la obesidad disminuye los niveles de adiponectina, lo cual fomenta la resistencia a la insulina y finalmente conduce a diabetes tipo 2.

Hay otra proteína de la célula grasa, llamada **resistina**, la cual desempeña un papel prominente en la causa de la diabetes y, en última instancia, la resistencia a la insulina. De hecho, además de diabetes, resistina promueven la enfermedad cardiovascular, hipertensión, accidentes cerebrovasculares, colesterol alto, cáncer, enfermedad hepática y asma.

Estas son algunas de las complicaciones metabólicas en la obesidad y la diabetes. Vamos a ver la influencia que tiene la socio-economía.

Aunque la obesidad ataca a niños de todos los estratos socioeconómicos, lo encontramos más entre los pobres, especialmente las personas de color (a menudo le dirá cualquier sociólogo, correlacionan los dos). Cuando los expertos investigaron el porque de este fenómeno, se dieron cuenta que están directamente ligados a cadenas de comida rápida omnipresentes dominando sus barrios. Uno de los atributos de estos restaurantes de comida rápida en estos vecindarios es, bueno, comida rápida. La comida es barata, sabrosa y densa en calorías, grasa y carbohidratos. Y para empeorar mas las cosas, los niños son animados o empujados a beber un "Big Gulp"-tipo azucarada bebida con cada comida, un refresco que contiene hasta 500 calorías de azúcar, 33% de lo que su cuerpo necesita en 24 horas.

Por otra parte, si consumen, digamos, una Big Mac con un big gulp, son otras 540 calorías. Agregale postre y papas fritas, esto obviamente excede la cantidad requerida para una comida sana y saludable.

Vamos a hablar del impacto socioeconómico. Mucha gente pobre necesitan trabajar dos trabajos para apenas sobrevivir o muchos luchan por salir adelante siendo padres de familia solteros. A menudo, los padres están demasiado cansados para arreglar comidas nutritivas por la noche, o los alimentos saludables no son fácilmente accesibles dentro de las limitaciones de tiempo o de una vida caótica y extremadamente angustiosa.

Con frecuencia, muchos niños pobres viven en comunidades con dispersión, tráfico rápido y colmado de pandillas. A menudo es inseguro jugar afuera después de la escuela. Los deportes organizados son caros (uniformes y cuotas), además se requiere transporte a las actividades de equipo. Así que, lamentablemente, los niños suelen estar en casa, pegado a la TV o el dispositivo electrónico. En vez de jugar deportes y juegos que quemen calorías al aire libre. Esto es la causa principal que conduce ala obesidad. Comer mucho y no hacer ejercicio.

Con el azúcar un componente principal de la dieta de un niño sedentario, un círculo vicioso metabólico estalla. Niveles de azúcar en la sangre aumentan, las páncreas producen menores cantidades de insulina causando que el apetito aumente.

Mientras tanto, el cerebro, puede ser engañado a señal de hambre en lugar de saciedad cuando el azúcar en la sangre primero subir y luego caer demasiado, demasiado rápido, después de una gran comida azucarada. Los niños terminan comiendo por comodidad, no por nutrición.

A pesar de datos contradictorios sobre este tema, es difícil negar que los niños que se exceden en las comidas altas en calorías basadas en azúcares y grasas se convierten en obesos, punto.

La Prediabetes, como su nombre lo indica, precede a menudo a la diabetes. ¿Las malas noticias acerca de la prediabetes? El paciente se tambalea al borde de su vida luchando contra la diabetes. ¿La buena noticia? Cuando esto es detectado temprano, la prediabetes puede ser arrestada al punto de que deje de girar fuera de control y se desarrolle en diabetes completo.

La prediabetes es un estado metabólico que generalmente se observa en personas obesas o con sobrepeso. A menudo estas personan muestran niveles de azúcar en la sangre que son normales, pero los niveles de insulina son elevados, estas son señales que las páncreas desesperadamente producen altos niveles de insulina para tratar de mantener el azúcar de sangre lo mas normal posible para compensar la resistencia a la insulina causada por esas células de grasa desagradables.

Para el paciente pre-diabético, vencer las probabilidades de desarrollar diabetes crónica no se requiero ser experto en matemáticas. Con el simple hecho de perder el 8% del peso corporal, reducir la ingestión de azúcar y calorías y hacer ejercicio, es posible prevenir el desarrollo de la diabetes tipo 2. Tómalo como si fuera un "triángulo de la salud": ejercicio, nutrición y descanso.

Uno creería que el hecho de entender sobre la pre-diabetes causaría un esfuerzo nacional para prevenir la obesidad, la cual es el espolón de muchos nuevos casos de la diabetes. Pongámonos a pensar en daño que se le hace a un niño que sube 40, 50 y hasta 60 libras de células graso-sas que contienen moléculas de proteínas múltiples que conducen a la diabetes, cáncer, enfermedades del corazón, cirrosis, artritis y angustia emocional. Esto es completamente criminal.

Pero es una lucha contra la corriente, teniendo en cuenta el poder de la industria azucarera y sus grupos de intereses. El color del dinero puede atraer incluso nuestras mejores instituciones educativas en cues-tionables investigaciones con resultados dudosos. En la década de 1960, por ejemplo, la Sugar Research Foundation patrocinó investigaciones por científicos de Harvard y les pagaron $50.000 por su participacion. El New England Journal of Medicine publicó los resultados en 1967. Como era de esperar, el informe de Harvard había minimizado otros estudios implicando azúcar como causa de enfermedad coronaria y la diabetes, echándole la culpa a las grasas y no ala azúcar.

¿Usted consigue lo que usted paga, correcto? Cual la lección aquí? cuidado con los estudios que son financiados por la industria de ali-mentos y comidas. Lo mismo va para el tabaco, licor y, bueno, lo diré, armas de fuego.

Cuando regrese de México en el año 2000, estaba decidido a ayudar a crear conciencia sobre la amenazadora epidemia de obesidad y dia-betes. Comencé en el lugar que sabía más, Santa Bárbara, California. La ciudad cuenta con un orgulloso patrimonio mexicano, con gran parte de su población de latinos viven en una sección llamada "el barrio este". Desafortunadamente, sin embargo, era difícil lugar para criar a niños saludables. Uno no podía caminar en el barrio con seguridad debido al alto tráfico y la ausencia de semáforos. Las pandillas iban en aumento, con balaceras de vez en cuando. La calle Milpas, que es la arteria prin-cipal del barrio, era (y sigue siendo) repleta de restaurantes de comida rápida. Tiendas de licores mostrando cartelones grandes de dulzuras a un lado de la caja registradora, tiendas del donas y pizzerías son puntos que componen el paisaje urbano.

Junto a la escuela Franklin, hay una escuela prescolar que va de kínder al sexto grado junto con una clínica de la comunidad donde se provee atención médica familiar. A un lado hay un jardín o parque comunitario al costado una clínica medica que provee servicios médicos básicos.

Recuerdos de mi experiencia como médico del cuerpo de paz en La Paz, Bolivia, 1969-1971, vinieron a la mente como considera establecer un programa de obesidad y bienestar en el barrio Este de Santa Bárbara. Aquí fue donde quise probar la hipótesis de que la obesidad infantil podría evitarse mediante la educación, esfuerzo comunitario y conciencia cultural. Al final, fue el apoyo y la motivación del alcalde de Santa Bárbara, SBCH programa de residencia, UC Santa Barbara, el Superintendente de las escuelas, los médicos locales y la Asociación Médica de California se sumaron a esta causa.

No nos equivoquemos, sin embargo. Aunque vivo y trabajo en Santa Bárbara, recursos como estos pueden ser movilizados para luchar contra la obesidad infantil en cualquier lugar.

En el año 2000, también fundé el centro de recursos de Diabetes (DRC) del Condado de Santa Bárbara, una corporación sin fines de lucro dedicada a reducir la alarmante epidemia de obesidad infantil en nuestra comunidad. Con el tiempo, recaudamos más de 1 millón de dólares de fundaciones caritativas, incluyendo the California Endowment, una Fundación de salud privada que trabaja para ampliar el acceso a cuidado de salud accesible, de alta calidad para las comunidades marginadas. La DRC trabajó sin problemas con sus socios para ayudar a cambiar el rumbo de la obesidad en la parte Este de nuestra comunidad..

Educación sobre los peligros a los niños y las familias de la obesidad infantil era prioridad número uno. Nos reunimos con líderes de la comunidad, el Principal de escuela de Franklin y el alcalde. Todos mostraban gran entusiasmo respecto a este proyecto.

Como era de esperar, sin embargo, había muchos que eran escépticos.

"Muchos creían que no se podía cambiar hábitos alimenticios o costumbres culturales o financiero que ya estaban bien plasmadas". Sabiendo esto y a través de nuestra relación con la escuela de Franklin y un director que apoyaron fuertemente a nuestro programa, se identificaron líderes de la comunidad natural y hacían Promotoras de Salud (promotores de salud) para ayudar a aclarecer cualquier diferencia que pudiera presentarse. Obtuvieron pequeñas recompenzas y eran bien educados acerca de los peligros de la obesidad como una causa de la diabetes, además de las funciones de nutrición y ejercicio para prevenir la enfermedad. Rápidamente entendieron el enorme peligro al bienestar de sus hijos y emprendieron con mucho afán sus nuevas funciones de promotoras de salud.

Muchas mujeres se convirtieron en "mamas sobreprotectoras," trabajando ferozmente para proteger la salud de sus hijos. Las mamas llevaban sus hijos de compras y aprendieron sobre alimentos procesados, refrescos y alimentos como saber como leer las en términos de calorías. Lamentablemente, comida fresca, organica o recién hecha eran extremadamente costosa, lo que es difícil para las familias a tomar esas decisiones saludables. Irónicamente, muchos papás y otros miembros de la familia trabajaban en los campos, recogiendo la mismas frutas y verduras que no podían consumir. Aún así, las mujeres compartían los conocimientos adquiridos a otros miembros de la comunidad y familias formaron "grupos de caminar a pie" para promover una salud mas sana.

La Escuela Franklin comenzó haciendo énfasis en educación física y especialistas llegaron a enseñar P.E. Los profesores todos participaron en clases aeróbicos después de la escuela para su propia salud y para servir como modelos para los estudiantes. Jardines de la escuela enriquecieron educación nutricional y más información sobre la ciencia.

Cuando comenzó el ano escolar, todos los niños se pesaron y su altura fue registrada. Con esta información, se calculó el índice de masa de corporal (IMC) de cada niño, una figura que utiliza una fórmula de la altura y el peso para definir y calcular sobrepeso, obeso y obeso mórbidos. Si un índice de masa corporal está en o por encima del 85% pero por debajo de los 95th, el niño tiene sobrepeso. Si un niño es mayor que el 95% , el niño es considerado obeso.

Esta base de datos nos tambaleó a todos. Cuarenta y cinco por ciento de los niños entrando al Kindergarten ya estaban con sobrepeso u obesidad. En K-6 grado, el 55% de ellos estaban con sobrepeso u obesidad, una tendencia horrible, trágica, de hecho muchos de esos niños, sin ninguna intervención, probablemente desarrollarían diabetes.

Recolectamos datos sobre los niños tres veces al año. Según avanzaba el programa, vimos reducciones estadísticamente significativas del

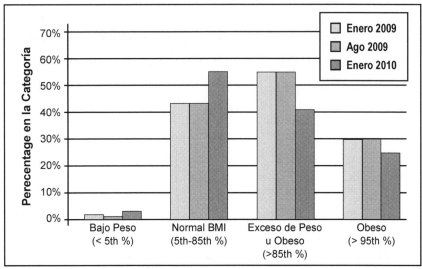

Figura 3: Todos los Niños

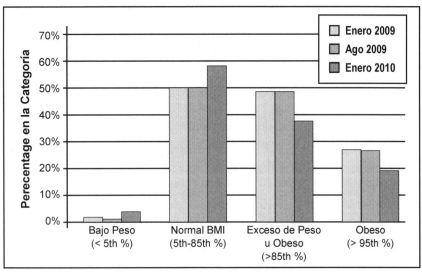

Figura 4: Todos los Niñas

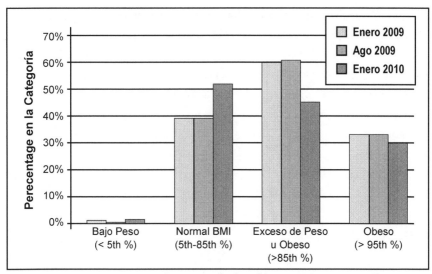

Figura 5: Todos los Chicos

índice de masa corporal por tres años seguidos. En Aquel entonces, el gobernador de California Arnold Schwarzenegger otorgo ala escuela Franklin una medalla de oro por sus esfuerzos, y la compañía de Blue Cross, junto con el gobernador, donó un gimnasio de lujo valorado en $100.000, equipado con máquinas adaptadas hacia el gimnasio de la juventud.

El DRC se rodeo de muchos voluntarios de UCSB, Westmont college y del colegio de Santa Bárbara .Su función era de documentar el índice de masa corporal, analizar datos, así como enseñar habilidades deportivas y de jardinería y hacer eventos para recaudación de fondos. Resultó una experiencia excelente, especialmente para los estudiantes de medicina, mostrándoles los retos de salud pública y de las raíces científicas de la obesidad. Muchos de estos voluntarios se beneficiaron al proveer más oportunidades de aprendizaje aparte de obtener cartas de recomendación para entrar a escuelas profesionales.

Una idea que nunca se implementó, pero todavía creo habría contribuido al programa de Franklin, fue una "receta de bienestar". En este modelo, los estudiantes obesos visitaría la clínica Franklin para evaluación médica, incluyendo análisis de sangre, para establecer la línea base lípidos, azúcar en la sangre y los niveles de insulina, además de un **CRP** (una prueba de proteína C reactiva detecta inflamación, de un evento agudo como una infección o de enfermedad crónica que requiere más pruebas para diagnosticar).

La prescripción de bienestar implicaría también formalmente los estudiantes en un programa de nutrición y actividad física (incluyendo podómetros para contar pasos y estimularlo a caminar). Promotoras de Salud ayudaría a las familias y los niños "mantienen el programa" y alentar a los padres para seguir con opciones de alimentación inteligente en casa. Con el tiempo, medimos y volvíamos a medir BMIs complementar los datos con el trabajo anual de la sangre. De manera que disminuía el BMI, probablemente se notaria una mejoría en los niveles de lípidos, los niveles de azúcar en la sangre y índices inflamatorios. Esa es mi hipótesis.

Cuando yo me enfermé, sin embargo, disolví el DRC que era sin fines de lucro e hizo la escuela Franklin, ya es una corporación sin fines de lucro, que recibiera todos los fondos dirigidos al DRC. Esto es realmente el modelo como opera los Peace corps. Educar, recaudar fondos, desarrollar programas de trabajan, luego pasarle todo a la Comunidad para que asuma todo el control.

Implementar un programa como este no es nada fácil, sobre todo a gran escala. Desafiará a cualquiera que trate de hacerlo, teniendo en cuenta la incesante fuerza de vientos políticos. Al igual que LeBron James tomándose un Sprite en televisión por dinero, la industria de comida rápida promueve vigorosamente campanas para preservar su control sobre las comunidades marginadas. Gritos como " Mantener fuera esos que regulan nuestras comidas fuera de nuestras vidas " y "Queremos nuestra libertad" socava cualquier intento de reducir la el consumo de comida chatarra y sus consecuencias devastadoras.

Cuando el alcalde Nueva York, Michel Bloomberg prohibió las grasas trans de los restaurantes de la ciudad porque causaban cáncer, la protesta al Gobierno de nuestras vidas era ensordecedoras. Cuando propuso reducir el tamaño de refrescos azucarados (a un "mero" 16 onzas), la industria de refrescos, que, a través de campañas políticas y relaciones públicas ya había derrotado a propuestas de soda-impuestos en todo el país, desafió los límites en la corte y ganó.

Incluso el senador Bernie Sanders, izquierdista, se opuso a imponer impuestos a las bebidas azucaradas para hacerlos menos disponible, porque, dijo, los pobres serian los mas afectados. No importa el hecho de que los niños puede beber el agua. No importa el escarpado impuesto sobre los cigarrillos. Nadie dice que cáncer daña a pobres porque son menos asequibles. ¿Dónde está la equidad, la educación, la conciencia? La obesidad mata al igual que los cigarros.

Cuando la primera dama Michelle Obama hizo de la obesidad infantil un pilar de su campaña educativa, los políticos la ridiculizaron. Ella sabia la magnitud de los problemas de la obesidad, especialmente entre las comunidades afro estadounidenses (y otros). Su influencia ayudo y mucho, pero sin el coraje y la voluntad política para abordar este problema de manera bipartidista, nuestros hijos se hacen más obesos, y nosotros vamos a necesitar ampliar nuestra unidad de diálisis, una vez más.

Además de promover la buena nutrición, la Sra. Obama había empujado ejercicio, la otra cara de la moneda de la obesidad. Dicho sin rodeos, Estados Unidos necesita una reforma nacional a promover más ejercicio. En caso de que esto no suceda, los pobres hábitos alimenticios y una vida sedentaria son una receta para un desastre fatal. Algunos de mis pacientes dicen que el ejercicio les ha salvado sus vidas tanto como sus preciosos trasplantes de riñón.

"Entiendo que ejercicio puede ser difícil," dice un paciente. "Tienes que conocer tu cuerpo y averiguar lo que funciona para ti. Si es caminar, camina. No trotar. Caminar rápido, subir ese ritmo cardíaco. Sudar. Busto de un grano. Empujar la sangre a través de todo su sistema vascular , desde las arterias mas grandes a los capilares más pequeños, alimentando tejido por tejido hasta los últimos rincones de cada órgano. El ejercicio no es sólo bueno para su corazón. Es bueno para cada parte de tu cuerpo. Sus ojos, los pulmones, las articulaciones, los músculos, el cerebro. Cualquier cosa que sea, hacer ejercicio es fundamental.

"Si usted tiene problemas de articulación, métase ala piscina. Nadar eleva su ritmo cardíaco y trabaja casi todos los músculos en su cuerpo. Lo sé, es frío, esta mojado, puede ser temprano por la mañana. ¿Y qué? ¿Quieres vivir? ¿Quieres ser sano? ¿Desea honrar a su donante de riñón? Entonces levantémonos de la cama o el sofá y a dale duro. Si no te gusta nadar, prueba ejercicios aqua-aeróbicos. Agua, especialmente la flotabilidad que ofrece, permite el ejercicio del no-peso-cojinete que puede hacer bien aunque uno este viejo.

"Sea lo que sea, párate, levántate y has ejercicio vigorosamente tres horas a la semana y síguelo haciendo. Para siempre. Hazlo parte de su vida como cepillarse los dientes. Lo sé. Es, a menudo muy duro. Por eso es un esfuerzo. Un sacrificio. Una manera de vivir mas saludable. Si se supone que es pura diversión, sino se llamaría diferente. Si se te dificultad, metete ala cabeza esto: "Si se puede, si puedo y puedo hacerlo", o "este dolor es sólo una debilidad que deja mi cuerpo. Y siempre recuerda: eres más fuerte de lo que piensas.

"Una vez que el ejercicio se convierte en una rutina de estilo de vida, usted crecerá adicto a ella, en el buen sentido. Vas a perderte cuando visites la abuela para el fin de semana o cuando un viaje de negocios interfiere con su rutina. Que es el cuerpo diciendo: ' me gusta estar sano; no olvide ejercerme pronto.'

"Y no se olvide el papel que el ejercicio tiene para reducir el estrés. Libera sustancias químicas como las endorfinas, que hacen que te sientes bien, 'alto del corredor,' por así decirlo. ¿Y lo que es mejor para el estrés que sentirse bien?

Otras maneras de reducir el estrés, tan frecuente en la vida frenética, alto voltaje de hoy, incluyen escribir, meditar, socializar (no aislarte) y pasar tiempo en la naturaleza. Una buena caminata en los parques, colinas o montañas nos hace pensar lo pequeño que somos , acompañados de nuestros temores y ansiedades.

Por eso, no es bueno preocuparse por detalles pequeños o cosas que uno no puede controlar lo cual puede conducir a más estrés que es completamente innecesaria la cual alimenta mas a otras enfermedades.

Soy consciente, como el refrán, que "grandes barcos gire lentamente", y que algunos pequeños programas alrededor de la nación ya se centran en la reducción de la obesidad. Ninguno, sin embargo, realmente incorporan el enfoque integral necesario para triunfar incluso modestamente. Así que, ¿cómo llegamos allí?

Propongo un cuerpo nacional de la salud, un programa similar al Peace corps que utiliza el poder y la inteligencia de los estudiantes voluntarios que pasan un año en el programa antes de ir a la Universidad. Aquí todos ganan. Voluntarios aprenden cuestiones de salud pública, medicina, sensibilidad cultural y la sociología de la pobreza, mientras que ayuda a frenar la creciente ola de obesidad infantil.

Seamos realistas: muchos jóvenes, incluso las cabezas más brillantes, a la Universidad socialmente no maduran lo suficiente para hacer su primer año significativo, si lo hacen en absoluto sin regresar a casa abrumado. Presión de grupo, fiestas, beber y sexo, y mucho menos la ansiedad de expectativas académicas y la soledad de salir de casa para el gran desconocido, pueden esperar hasta un año.

Así es, un año, un año pasado en un programa de cuerpo nacional de la salud, un año de público (modestamente dotado) servicio para estimular la madurez, desarrollan un sentido de propósito, incluso profundizar en futuras carreras. El camino conduce a la sociología, la antropología, la medicina o el servicio público, un año de servicio del cuerpo de salud pudo vencer el valor de estar aturdido en una clase de 800 enseñadas por un estudiante graduado, o tropezar confuso en el primer paso de la vida independiente. No hay ninguna magia acerca de cómo iniciar el colegio a los 18 años. Diecinueve funciona igual de bien, mejor aún, en la mayoría de los casos.

La tecnología actual parece estar obsesionada con el entrenamiento de la próxima generación de jóvenes emprendedores. Énfasis en ingeniería, negocios y programación informática ha suplantado los compromisos a las artes y las Humanidades, elementos esenciales para una vida plena y una sociedad plena y desarrollada. ¿No sería genial si mentes jóvenes, mentes excepcionales prestarían su inteligencia para resolver los problemas que amenazan a nuestros hijos y nuestro sistema de salud, aunque solo por un año?

Con la Presidencia de Obama aparentemente una memoria distante, impulso y entusiasmo acerca de prevención de la obesidad serán temas seguramente olvidados. El tema caliente se va evaporando y con el tiempo se oscurece la visión. Como la comodidad de un sillón reclinable que se siente bien ahora, pero que lentamente te matará, tu estado psíquico, es como que es mas fácil batallar con malas noticias, malas políticas y malos resultados a la estera de lucha. Me preocupan las familias, especialmente los niños, que sólo conseguirán ser más gordos. Y créanme, una nación crónicamente enfermiza siempre se mantendrá marginada.

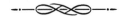

Chapter 17

My Odyssey of Stress and How I Ended It

While writing this book and reflecting on my own journey, I undertook what I call "stress mapping" to see where I collected the stress that later erupted into lung cancer and other problems. Of course, stress was probably not the only contributor, but I'm convinced it was a major trouble-maker. To understand my health—and I recommend you apply the same stress-mapping technique in your life—I needed to know where and how I fell into the stress trap even if it was self-induced.

I realized it began in 1964, when I started studying medicine. I was basically poor, had no source of transportation, no knowledge of what healthy food looked like, or any experience cooking. By November, the first of many snowstorms hit Syracuse, and the sun hardly shone again until spring. I drove myself so hard that, by the end of that first year, I already felt negative physical effects from sitting for countless hours in library stacks, where I memorized the entire human anatomy. By spring, friends and I got together to play basketball on Saturdays, which was a joy. I felt rejuvenated and ready to vigorously hit the stacks again, for biochemistry and other sundry disciplines.

With a rear-view mirror, however, it's easy to see errors I made. Because I didn't cook for myself I had little understanding of healthy eating, and could only afford basic starchy foods, processed meats, and casseroles. My diet, devoid of fiber and green vegetables, played a major role laying the groundwork for diverticulosis later in life—inflammation and ultimate (serious) infection of diverticula, formed from a weakness in the colon wall resembling micro-balloons. I was chronically constipated throughout medical school due to my unhealthy lifestyle. Strain on the colon from trying to move my bowels, combined with sleep deprivation and a GI tract that felt abandoned, led to my early diverticular disease.

I had charted a super-ambitious course of study, then created a wild, feverish, unsustainable pace. I had little choice if I wanted to achieve my dream of becoming a doctor. I was young. I felt invincible, almost immortal (which I considered heroic), as though I was doing a "white-knight" thing. Turns out, it was almost a "goodnight" thing, because I'd inadvertently, unknowingly, planted the seeds of illness. I completed medical school and residency, but the sneaky thing about stress and physical disease is that it can be cumulative, laying coiled and dangerous like a snake in your system for years.

Nearly a decade later, my wife, Leslie and I were driving from Santa Barbara to San Diego to help our son, then a UC San Diego student, move to new housing. That's when abdominal pain began, at first mild but then steadily worsening. It became so painful, I had to switch places and let Leslie drive. The following week, we helped our daughter Danielle move from our Santa Barbara home to her dorm at Northwestern University in Evanston, Illinois, a three-day drive. This time, I suffered severe abdominal pain and knew something was seriously wrong.

I was distracted, however, more focused my daughter's stress than my own. She'd made the University swim team as a walk-on, but nervous that she had to compete on a team of scholarship athletes, some of them record-holders in high school. Plus, she was moving far from home for the first time.

I worried about her. Danielle had suffered from minimal-change disease as a child and was still prone to relapses associated with massive swelling and protein loss in her urine. I was reminded, later, about Mary's story, when she was erroneously diagnosed with minimal-change disease only to have a more serious diagnosis of focal sclerosis. Before I gained a firm understanding of Danielle's illness, I had recurrent dreams of donating a kidney to her.

When we arrived back in Santa Barbara, a CT scan showed that I was suffering from acute diverticulitis. By then, I had lost weight, was continuing to lose weight, and felt fatigued. Doctors prescribed antibiotics, but appetite loss and weakness persisted.

Ironically, I had recently seen a hospitalized patient who also had severe diverticulitis. She had developed a fistula (connection between organs) between her bladder and colon, a life-threatening situation. She developed sepsis, renal failure and died! Later, I treated Ed, whose story is highlighted in this book. He developed diverticulitis while he still had a transplanted kidney. Ed had to have a portion of his colon removed and required an external bag, called a colostomy, to collect his bowel movements.

Though familiar today with cases in which diverticulitis has fatal consequences, in those days I didn't do much about it except take antibiotics. No surprise, really, that I didn't improve. A major part of the problem, I realize now, was that I pushed myself to go to the office to see patients, take calls, visit hospital patients. In retrospect, I should have done what I always counsel my patients to do—listened to my body. I should have rested. How many of you are like that right now? Take my advice, from one who's been there: rest if you need to! In the long run, far more time, energy, and clear thinking emerge from a healthy body than one wracked with chronic fatigue.

Perhaps from a misplaced sense that I was indispensable to my patients' health, or maybe driven by an unrealistic work ethic, I didn't listen to my body, even though it screamed, "Slow down." I ignored the Biblical reminder, "Physician, heal thyself," and blindly pushed on.

A vicious circle can begin as you try to power through work and life, even though your subconscious knows something is wrong and you need to rest. Whether you know it or not, stress is pressing down, eroding your ability to make sound decisions, along with so many other negative consequences.

Fear can creep in because you know deep-down this is not working, and you need serious medical attention. For a scholarly discussion of this concept, I recommend Dr. Gabor Mate's bestselling book, translated into 15 languages and read in 5 continents, *"When the Body Says NO, Exploring the Stress-Disease Connection."*

My stress level continued rising because a little, annoying voice kept telling me I had a serious problem that would likely require surgery. Simultaneously, I suffered what patients everywhere suffer: lack of a clear path to healing. Did I really need surgery, which could be quite serious, or would antibiotics alone "cure" me? I chased my tail, trying to assess my choices and pick the best path forward.

On one hand, I thought, the medical team wanted to "cure" me with antibiotics alone to spare me the surgery, even though literature I read suggested surgery was the treatment of choice when the antibiotics stubbornly fail their mission. I found myself stuck in an ironic quagmire: I suffered terrible stress over a decision about a malady that was most likely abetted by stress, poor diet, and insufficient exercise from years earlier.

If that wasn't enough, a short time earlier my business partner Dr. Tom Allyn and I had scrambled to borrow money from family and a bank to develop the Santa Barbara Artificial Kidney Center. This was a big financial risk, with no "given" that it would succeed or ably compete against a large corporation already supplying dialysis services to the community. We pursued the idea not out of financial confidence, but because we were committed to supplying better services to some very sick patients who needed a personal touch. The single company running a dialysis unit in Santa Barbara was a controlling, inflexible firm seemingly more interested in bottom-line earnings than superior patient care. We were determined to provide an alternative.

So, beside anciety about my medical condition, I stayed up nights worrying about a risky decision that might generate suffocating debt for my family if it failed. Stress! Stress! I often told my patients that once they identified their sources of stress, they should immediately act to diminish them. Thankfully, this time I followed my own advice and had a long talk with my accountant, who assured me the business risk I was taking wasn't foolish.

Nonetheless, I still paid a price for the self-induced stress I'd created over the years. One morning, I awoke before sunrise and went to the bathroom. I'd lost over 15 pounds and was feeling generally miserable due to my poor, declining health. The moment urine flowed I screamed with agonizing pain. Instantly, I thought of my patient who developed kidney failure and sepsis, then died with diverticulitis. The thought stunned me. I convinced myself that I was headed down the same road. It starts with an overwhelming infection caused by stool from the colon entering the bladder and traveling into the kidneys and bloodstream. As I mentioned, its pathology can range from mild to fatal. The pain in my abdomen suddenly grew insanely intense as my inflamed colon went into spasm. It felt fatal at the time.

I headed to the hospital. A surgeon ordered studies to visualize my colon. As I waited for the exam, supine on a cold, hard, metal table, frightening thoughts gripped my mind. Then a brisk, grim-looking technician entered the room. With little regard or recognition that I was a sick, frightened, patient, he went about his job, placing a tube into my rectum, while briefly explaining that material will flow into the colon while x-rays were taken.

I recount this personal moment not for attention or sympathy, but to let you know that I have been where you are now or may be in the future. It may seem like you are alone in what you endure—humiliated, confused, angry—but you aren't alone. Sure, in an existential sense, nobody but you knows your personal joy, sadness, or pain. But together we can change the medical system from an impersonal conveyor belt to one in which patients are universally treated with respect and a caring hand. It's happening in some hospitals and clinics, but they are the exception to the norm of overly conservative values, rushed treatments, sterile relationships with caregivers, and a pursuit of dollars over dignity.

For the second time within a few hours, I was alone in agony, screaming in unmitigated pain as a barium-like liquid reached my narrowed and inflamed sigmoid colon. Nobody came into the room to assess my situation, let alone try to comfort me. The pain was so intense I started screaming profanities and removed the tube to stop the flow and the pain it was causing. Finally, the technician came in, showing no emotion other than his displeasure over my language. Had I been able to get out of bed, I might have given him something else to add to his displeasure. But I was helpless. Helpless and unspeakably miserable.

During times like these, medical staff (hopefully some are reading this) can provide incredible comfort to patients. A soft, comforting word, especially combined with the human element—a soft touch or soft rubbing on the arm—can do the trick. I've seen it. I teach it. I embrace it.

But this time? No so much. After my rather colorful "request" that he *do something,* this fellow administered some strong pain-killing meds. My wife Leslie, who was far down the hallway, heard my outcry and ran quickly to my side, holding my hand, providing the care I needed, while no physician or nurse bothered stopping by.

(After this was over, I made my displeasure about how I was treated very clear to hospital administrators. Anyone should do this if they feel mistreated. On the other hand, it's important to tell administrators and caregivers when someone does a great job. It's easier to complain than compliment, but both forms of feedback are essential for clinical administrators.)

The Humanitarian

The night before surgery to assess and repair my damaged colon, Dr. Steve Hosea, an infectious-disease specialist and director of our residency program, visited me. He wore a big smile and after talking a bit, placed his hands on the sides of my head and held them there for several seconds. When he left, I felt like he'd transferred positive energy into me. That human touch alone felt reassuring and, in its way, incredibly healing—especially since I'd been told, in clinical terms, that because of my tremendous weight loss, I might have cancer. In fact, doctors warned me that during surgery they may have to perform a colostomy.

Deep fear and more stress!

My wife and Dr. Steve Hosea's visit got me through it. My surgeon, Dr. Lang, did a masterful job of removing very sick intestine, avoiding the need for a colostomy. When I awoke from the surgery, I was told it went well—no colostomy and my bladder would heal. I could have cried, I think maybe I did.

After being discharged, some stress abated but some remained, and I did not do a good job of dealing with it. I was already thinking about obligations to patients, my partner, and other nephrologists with whom I worked. I knew I had to gain back 15 pounds and recover energy I had lost. But, instead of taking on a positive attitude and getting excited about healing, I immediately expected top performance from myself and judged my own lack of energy harshly. Today, that seems downright silly, even idiotic, and an obvious blueprint for more health problems. But, I was so caught up in life and the need to achieve certain goals, I couldn't see it then. I became a living example of how excessive self-criticism, a lack of "mindfulness," and not taking time to rest and find joy in life, can bring you down, no matter who you are or what you do. We must be gentler on ourselves.

I returned to work, and surprise! I awoke one morning with yet another physical problem, this time, a left lower abdominal pain. Stress had caused it indirectly, yet now it was causing me even more stress. Anxiety gnawed at my stomach. What was this, what more could happen? A complication from the diverticulitis surgery?

Nope, this time an x-ray revealed a kidney stone. The chronic dehydration and weight loss I'd experienced during my illness predisposed kidney-stone formation. It seemed that there was no end to health issues I faced. As soon as I addressed one, another slipped silently into the queue. What I didn't realize (and this should rank as an elemental part of societal understanding and physicians' curriculum) was the stress I constantly experienced was attacking my immune system, and now it no longer defended me, but was attacking me instead.

The stone was stubborn and would not pass, despite drinking of copious amounts of fluid. Kidney stones, as you probably know, are quite painful, causing a knifelike ache each time the body tries to move it down the ureter. I required a procedure called lithotripsy, which uses ultrasonic shock waves to break up the stone, which then passes in the urine as pulverized fragments, not completely without pain itself. Finally, the stone exited my body as sludge in the urine.

Looking back, this would have been (another) time for me to relax, practice yoga, learn to stay present-centered and allow abundant happiness and excitement into my life. I didn't, and was about to pay another significant price.

Less than a year later, central vision began decreasing in my left eye. Over time, it got worse. An ophthalmologist diagnosed my problem as central serous retinopathy, a condition poorly understood, but highly associated with stress. My disease was near the macula (at the center of the retina), which made it untreatable using the laser technology of the time. Gradually, I went blind in that eye.

Devastated, I swirled in emotional turmoil. Seemed like a reservoir of unnecessary stress, fueled by years of pushing myself too hard, breaking treaties with my immune system, had come back to haunt me again. In retrospect, it was all so unnecessary.

And yet, I still hadn't figured that out. I continued working at a break-neck pace, believing my patients needed me every moment. And the more I worked, the more patients I accumulated, abetting a vicious cycle that was wrecking my body. As a man, I derived my worth, my value on the planet, from being a father, husband, and doctor. I hadn't yet connected with the higher purpose of just being and loving—not an easy thing for men to learn, especially in modern America.

Had I learned my lesson yet? Nope. A couple of years later, I awoke one day to mild discomfort in both hands. Over time, the pain gradually worsened. I grew fatigued and began feeling miserable again. I also developed a new outbreak of psoriasis, a skin condition associated with small, scaly, reddish patches found especially on extensor surfaces of the knees and elbows. (I first suffered from this as a medical student. Though the disease was mild, these patches became bright red before a challenging school exam.) Fast-forward, my rheumatologist diagnosed the psoriatic arthritis when an x-ray of my hand revealed destruction of outer bone tissue called the cortex.

No drugs prescribed effectively reduced the pain or improved my energy level. In fact, as drugs often do, they began creating problems of their own. My liver enzymes became elevated, due to hepatotoxicity caused by a drug methotrexate, used for this condition. My joints still ached, and fatigue became debilitating.

After making hospital rounds and seeing patients in the office one day, I slumped into bed, lethargic and fatigued. Lying there, I contemplated what condition my condition was in. Could I continue my heavy workload, be an able partner to my wife, a dad to three active children, and meet financial demands? In addition, we were still developing the Santa Barbara Artificial Kidney Center, which was growing rapidly due to an epidemic of diabetes and kidney failure.

I was still clueless. I hadn't learned how to deflect stress or to turn it into a positive challenge. So, it persisted, and I remained on the merry-god-round of stress and illness.

Finally, an injectable drug called Embrel became available to treat inflammatory arthritis—good news because after only a few injections, my pain abated and my energy level rose. The bad news was that by the time I'd developed psoriatic arthritis, my immune system was severely compromised.

Embrel was the first of a new class of medicines that works by blocking an important part of the cytochrome pathway, facilitated by the immune system. One component, called tumor necrosis factor alpha, was elevated in my blood and responsible for my joint pain and systemic weakness. When Embrel blocks this factor, arthritis improves, but the drug dramatically suppresses the immune system. Superimposed on an already debilitated immune system, it was a perfect storm for developing cancer.

Phil Mickelson, a professional golfer who has psoriatic arthritis, was on television at the time, delivering a testimonial based on his experience about the benefits of this drug. At the end of the ad came a chilling warning that this class of drugs can cause severe infection or cancer. I didn't pay enough attention—or didn't want to pay attention—to that warning.

For years following, I injected myself with Embrel, and later a newer version, injected less often, called Humira. My arthritis remained in remission, but, in 2013, I developed a lesion on my tongue. My doctors believed it was related to the use of these drugs and was either cancer or an infection. More stress.

Lung Cancer and a Life-Saving Revelation

I planned yet another surgery. Because of it, I was scheduled to have a chest x-ray before the operation at UCLA. A discussion with a head-and-neck surgeon proved a bit scary, as he outlined possible outcomes. If a large portion of my tongue needed to be resected because of cancer, I was in serious trouble—radiation, chemotherapy, impaired speech, impaired eating, and who-knows-what-else. On a scale of 1 to 10, my stress level hit 11.

Surgery revealed a chronic infection, not cancer. That was the good news. A week later, however, surgeons removed a lobe of my left lung. Like a bell-ring at a carnival hammer-swing, my stress hit an all-time high, completely off the charts.

Nobody can point to a single cause of my lung cancer, but I believe stress dating back to my quest to become a doctor, plus medical residency with inhuman work hours leading to chronic sleep deprivation, eating poorly on the run, and practicing a difficult specialty tending to the sickest of sick patients, sowed the seeds.

Recovering from lung surgery proved a godsend. This time, I was so weak and debilitated I had no choice but to rest. I cannot describe a magic moment, a book, or inspirational quote that sent me toward a deeper understanding of the complete melding of body and mind. I just know it happened. As I slowly recovered, I became convinced of what I had always suspected: a close tie between emotional and physical health. I got excited because I instinctively knew I was headed in the right direction. I began mentally stress-mapping my own life, lying in bed, healing in a more powerful way than I ever could have imagined. A light flickered, and I "got it." I finally understood where lay the key to my own health—it was in my own head, in a rekindled belief that relaxation and accepting myself and the world in a loving way were the not-so-secret keys to my transformation.

I am now healthy, for the first time since I can remember.

No matter the illness you or a loved one might suffer, there are ways to triumph, especially with rapidly unfolding new treatments and cures, and especially if you keep your end of the bargain with your immune system. One great benefit of a low-stress lifestyle: it makes for easy, comfortable, compassionate, loving, and caring good times—a positive, upward spiral if ever there was one.

These days, I've slowed down to write this book, I don't take many calls, I eat healthfully, exercise, and practice yoga. I spend time with my wife Leslie, my three children and seven grandchildren. The stress that shackled my life has noticeably decreased, and my energy and zest have returned.

Benjamin Disraeli, former prime minister of the United Kingdom, once said, "There is no education like adversity." From it, you can grow, gain personal insights, and learn what it takes not only to overcome, but to live a joyful, healthy life. Pieces of the puzzle often hide in plain sight. The challenge is to find ones that best fit you and provide the best balance for your body and soul.

Mind-Body Relations Should Reside at the Heart of Western Medicine

Academics whose work stems from outcome-based research that relies strictly on the mathematics of statistics, have said, "The enemy of science is subjectivity." But, what if subjectivity already exists in deciding when to pursue science to prove or disprove certain beliefs? I recently read chapters on stress, immunology, immunology of the brain, and rheumatology, including connective-tissue autoimmune diseases such as lupus and rheumatoid arthritis, in the latest Harrison textbook of medicine. (*Harrison's Principles of Internal Medicine,* originally written by Tinsley R Harrison and published in the 1950s' has long been considered one of the "Bibles" of Western medicine.)

Reading it was like swimming through wet cement, because pathways the immune system utilizes to ultimately prevent disease are incredibly complex. Laudably, scientists now understand myriad reactions taking place in lymphocytes, our thymus-derived immune cells, though their intricacy is mind-boggling, to say the least. The endpoint is a protein called a cytokine. Eighty-One of these play a central role in regulating immune and inflammatory responses. (Don't fret the science too much—just thought you might enjoy more "nerdy" aspects of how our bodies work.)

I mention cytokines, however, for a reason—to point out how the medical system has been sluggish to understand the infinite value of the mind-body relationship. Physicians trained in highly-academic institutions find it exhilarating to be asked on morning rounds, "What are the cytokines that comprise the interleukin cascade, and in what order do they appear in a response to an inflammatory lesion?" Eager students like me jump to answer, in large part because knowing information like this gives them, and physicians a (false) sense of control over miserable diseases like lupus and other autoimmune illnesses. Everybody—students and faculty alike—feels brilliant. But smugness doesn't make patients feel better, cure disease, or hasten recovery. Rarely, in fact, do medical students or doctors discuss trickier parts of a patient's history, especially possible connections between stress and an illness like systemic lupus.

Ask most physicians why the "scientific method" (including review of evidence subject to specific principles of reasoning) has not been applied to this question, they'll typically frown and tell you, "Because it's irrelevant to researchers." The "subjective bias" of determining the amount of stress a patient has experienced, they might contend, makes it an "unusable" variable in Western medicine. This is why most physicians take a near-dismissive approach to considering the mind-body connection. (There exist, however, glimmers of hope. Increasingly, some doctors, albeit a minority, are working to break down old barriers, old mindsets.)

But don't misunderstand. We should appreciate and continue relying upon the intricate, highly technical, scientific approach to patient care as well. Consider, for example, the pharmaceutical industry and brilliant researchers who've discovered and engineered miraculous drugs that allow us to transplant a kidney into patient from a donor with a different blood type—the so-called "ABO-incompatible match." The same folks, same researchers, same surgeons, and care-givers that helped ease my pain and save my life.

A scientist, however, should always remain open to a panoply of healing methods, even if mechanisms by which they work are not fully understood (some might say acupuncture fits here, though evidence strongly suggests it can help stimulate the body's self-healing capacities). If physicians' goal is helping our patients live the healthiest lives possible, we need to listen not only to their words when taking medical histories, but also their "music." To me, the connection between prolonged stress and development of myriad diseases seems obvious. The time has come for more medical practitioners to acknowledge this possibility and factor it into prevention, diagnosis, treatment, and therapy. Trusting your instincts and intuition may prove as valuable as the procedure you order or prescription you write.

If we look at literature from the psychiatric discipline, we find an entirely different story. Dr. Gabor Mate's book, *"When the Body Says No"* (noted earlier) explores the role of prolonged exposure to noxious stressors as a causative factor in disease. He concludes that diseases such as lupus, rheumatoid arthritis, cancer, and multiple sclerosis directly relate to prolonged stressful experiences. His work and that of many others in his field arrive at the same conclusions. When he discusses causes of lung cancer, for example, he indicates that many physicians point the finger at smoking. He asks, "Why do only a relatively small number of smokers get cancer?" His answer? Lung cells in a smoker are predisposed to develop cancer, but something needs to weaken the immune system, allowing the bad cells to get an upper hand. Stress seems like the likeliest culprit. Think about people who smoke. Are they not among the most stressed-out folks you know?

Television personality Bill Moyers wrote a book called *Healing and The Mind* and organized it around the worthiness of a journey to learn about the "remarkable union of mind, body, and spirit that is the human being." He wanted to know how our thoughts and feelings influence our health, and how they relate to our minds. He spoke with scientists engaged in the emerging field of psychoneuroimmunology, bringing together psychiatrists, neurologists, immunologists, and endocrinologists, all seeking to understand the mind-body relationship. After returning from China, where he studied ancient Eastern approaches to healing, he concluded that, "We in the West, do not have to give up our proven resources to appropriate the best that another culture has to offer; here well may be the crucible where East meets West to forge a new source of healing."

Moyers interviewed Dr. Thomas Delbanco, professor of medicine at Harvard University, who starts by saying, "I hope I'm addressing both the body and the mind, but they are so intertwined it's hard for me to differentiate. I know more about the body than the mind. It's probably easier to study and that's what we learned in medical school—95 percent body, 5 percent brain. But I'll tell you, once you're in practice and taking care of real people, it becomes more like fifty-fifty."

Dr. Candace Pert, PhD, a world-class scientist and chief of Brain Biochemistry of the Clinical Neuroscience Branch at the National Institute of Mental Health, helped augment our understanding of the complex relationship between brain and body. That relationship, if you look at its complexities, is nothing short of fascinating. For example, much of the intimate communication between mind and body is mediated through strands of amino acids strung together to form proteins called peptides. Receptors for these peptides exist not only in the brain, but in almost every cell of the body. Think of them and their receptors as "chemicals of emotion" found in parts of the brain that mediate emotion. They control, for example, the opening and closing of blood vessels in your face. They allow body systems to talk to each other. In real life, the brain and the immune system use so many of the same molecules to communicate with each other that we're beginning to see perhaps the brain is not simply "up here," connected by nerves to the rest of the body. We're discovering that cells of the immune system constantly filter through the brain and can lodge there. When scientists discovered energy-laden hormones called endorphins in the brain, which cause euphoria and pain relief, everybody could handle that. But, when they discovered they were in your immune system, too, that fact was denied for years—more ignorance of the mind-body connection.

These peptides determine whether a virus can successfully enter a cell or not, and therefore determine a physical illness or not. Emotional fluctuations and stress directly influence the probability that an organism (us) will get sick or stay well.

Sadly, I have not seen hard data to prove a statistically significant cause and effect, or at least none that have commanded the attention of academic physicians. This material is not taught in medical school, perhaps in part because scientific data on large groups of people with high-stress histories, people who go on to develop immune-system diseases, have not been collected. In a psychiatry course in medical school, we learned the basics about major psychiatric illnesses such as schizophrenia, bipolar disease, depression, and anxiety. Although important information, it serves a limited purpose in daily medical practice.

I know, I know. Of course, we need to screen patients for serious psychiatric disorders, but we'd all benefit from discussing the mind-body connection and the latest data explaining it. In some progressive medical schools with integrative medicine programs, the mind-body connection is incorporated into the curriculum, but acceptance by the medical community continues to lag. Only when young physicians accept the high probability that noxious events occurring for long periods of time in people's lives present significant variables linked to severe illnesses, will a concerted effort to check these stressors integrate into how we practice medicine. Put simply, reducing their intensity through a variety of methods, early enough to prevent catastrophic disease, should complement the canons of treatment advanced by today's doctors.

The disconnect between mind doctors and body doctors in 21st century medicine remains shocking and absurd. It's time to emulate Albert Einstein's vision of a unifying theory of the nature of the universe, but in our case, the nature of the human body. The brain communicates with and controls every organ system in our body through complex chemicals and hormones it synthesizes and sends to other organs that respond in specific ways. Then it receives input from organs like the kidney, liver, heart, intestines, and, of course, the immune system. Physicians of every specialty should be open to obvious interactions and consequences of this organic "we're all in it together" relationship.

Little of what I've learned about connections between our emotional state, our immune system, and the state of our physical health, came from books. It came from pain, sickness, and, finally, knowledge that if we don't help our immune system take care of us, we will need doctors—many of whom don't understand or value our emotional needs. So, we need to stick to the bargain we have with our immune systems. They're the best doctors in the world and will take care of us if we give them a chance.

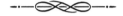

Reflections

Recovering from my own surgery, I was drawn to my most challenged patients because they inspired me with their undaunted determination to overcome adversity. Reflecting on their complex histories, it also appeared that the convoluted twists and turns, the ups and downs, of their journeys might inspire people suffering from complex diseases or facing similar, seemingly insurmountable challenges.

They tell the tale of human resolve trumping catastrophic illness. More broadly considered, their courage to own their situations and persevere apply to overcoming all manner of adversity, from abuse to addiction, disease to divorce, bullying to bankruptcy. In this way, their tales are universal.

While I purposely chose to share dramatic stories, many of my patients experienced far simpler, successful outcomes. Some have had their original kidney transplants for up to 30 years, without major complications. The notable cases, however, speak more directly to the capability and triumph of the human will.

And though these stories can sadden a reader, I hope their positive outcomes outweighed the pain endured (for the patients *and* for you). If you asked them if they'd change any aspect of their journeys, they'd likely say, "Nope, I would have made the same decisions." For them it was a native, internal determination, a choice of life—a real life, with real reasons to live—over death, either sudden or by "a thousand cuts," conveyed by immutable chronic disease or the slow, grinding debilitation of health maintenance.

Their stories also reflect the triumph of modern medicine. In some cases, the timeline of patients' battles coincided with medical advances that ultimately cured them. Mick, who had four kidney transplants, benefitted from advances in dialysis, transplant surgical techniques, and a revolution in immunotherapy during his 37-year medical odyssey.

"Stick and stay to make it pay," he tells me, was his mantra—words to live by for overcoming whatever ails you. Or, as Winston Churchill famously said, "If you're going through hell, keep going." The patients in this book all went through hell and, in one form or another, made it through to a better life.

The theme that we can overcome the penetrance of bad genes that predispose us to developing diabetes, autoimmune disease, or cancer by implementing lifestyle changes, weaves a lighted path through this book. Simply put, a steady measure of common sense, resolve, and self-control can save lives. The sciences of epigenetics and psychoneuroimmunology confirm this as fact, not just belief. Consider the role of stress in your life and the lives of loved ones and friends. In that sample alone, you'll likely find anecdotal evidence of my assertion. Stress kills, just like obesity, and both are on an epic run that, to be reversed, will require unmatched resolve from patients, doctors, and politicians, all the way to Pennsylvania Avenue.

I continue to believe that it can be accomplished. Today's Franklin School experiment can be tomorrow's nationwide awakening. With patience, perseverance, and education about the "why" to make radical behavioral changes, and by embracing healthy living, people will find the "how."

I hope that you enjoyed this book and, along with the work of others, heed the advice to treat the causes of our great 21st-century epidemics—stress, obesity, and sedentary behavior—before they overwhelm you. Over time, we'll make progress on the medical and holistic fronts, too. As it's been with monsters like smallpox and bubonic plague, deaths from diabetes, heart disease, and kidney failure will ultimately decline.

Finally, I share with you some thoughts from the first several weeks after my cancer surgery, when I couldn't escape thinking about time and purpose in life. I visualized my life as a large, stained-glass mosaic, filled with pieces of varying size, shape, and color—reflections and reminders of the pieces making up the entirety of a life's work and experience. I could see that and there was still space to fill more pieces over the coming years, but an uncertainty about accomplishing this loomed dark and shadowy. Of course, life is uncertain with no warranties. It's a crap-shoot. I knew it then as I know it now. So, be grateful every morning when you can get out of bed, all your senses intact, take a deep, effortless breath, and greet another day. Time, and only time, remains our most precious resource.

As I lay in bed, debilitated and depressed, I wondered if I had time left to fill in those last stained-glass pieces of my life's mosaic, or would the mosaic be left unfinished? That proved a pivotal moment that allowed me to revisit the struggles of my brave patients and their unwillingness to surrender. From their energy, love of life, and courage, plus the heroism of people who came forward to donate kidneys, I drew resolve to fight on, get well, and find new purpose and pathways in life, though different than the one I may have originally charted.

I still get great satisfaction seeing patients in my office, but I see fewer of them, freeing me from the stress-inducing constraints of time. This allows me to give them all the time they need. Time spent with patients, and the quality of that time, not the number of patients seen, are what now define me as a physician. I allow the time patients need to tell me in detail what ails them. I pay even closer attention to physical exams because I know there aren't several anxious patients in the sitting room waiting to see me. My cancer battle, as difficult as it was, gave me this new perspective, a new way to experience the joy of practicing medicine.

When asked if I would still choose doctoring and whether I'd do it differently, I say "yes" and "yes." It's been a great privilege to have won the trust of patients for something so precious as their safety, wellbeing, and life. Even if I'd known the path to becoming a physician would be as stressful and demanding as it's been, I would have chosen it—with one exception. I would have drawn a line in the sand about work hours. I needed time, my time, to run, move, see my kids more often, be a better listener, give my wife more support, and grow into a complete human being.

Patients idolize doctors and unrealistically believe we're superhuman (part of why I rarely wear a lab coat). Doctors, unconsciously or not, buy into this myth and acquire a persona of indispensable, celestial beings—a hubris that leads to hasty diagnoses, lousy beside manners, arrogance, and self-destructive behavior.

Many great physicians can do this job. I've learned, however, that aspiring to greatness may not require sacrificing precious personal time to live and grow. It does, however, require attention to detail and to the humanity that binds us all. In the end, balancing all this in an ever-changing, complex universe may be the greatest aspiration of all.

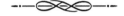

Glossary

Acidosis Too much acid in the blood directly related to the failure of the kidneys to excrete it

Adenosine A drug used to bring a heart back into normal rhythm. It may also be used to test the heart for coronary artery disease

Adipocytes Cells specialized for the storage of fat, found in connective tissue

Adiponectin A protein hormone which is involved in regulating glucose levels as well as fatty acid breakdown

Adrenal glands Small organs sitting on top of each kidney that secrete among other hormones, aldosterone which causes the kidney to retain salt and water

Adult Onset Diabetes Also called type 2 diabetes, results in 95% of all cases of diabetes in the world and is the most common cause of kidney failure

Albumen A protein that lives in the blood stream and is synthesized in the liver. When it appears in the urine it signals kidney disease

ANA test An antinuclear antibody test that measures the amount and pattern of antibodies in your blood that work against your own body (autoimmune reaction)

Anemia A low red-blood-cell count with myriad causes. When the kidneys fail to synthesize erythropoietin during the course of kidney failure, the patient develops the anemia of kidney failure

Anti-Diuretic Hormone (ADH) A protein stored and synthesized in the brain, released when a person is dehydrated. Kidneys respond to its release by retaining water and concentrating urine

Aneurysm Weakness in the wall of a large blood vessel, frequently caused by hypertension, which leads to a ballooning of the vessel, which, in turn, can rupture and lead to life-threatening blood loss

Angiotensin 2 A powerful agent that causes severe constriction of blood vessels and subsequent hypertension. Failing kidneys indirectly increase this protein

Antibody A protein synthesized by the immune system in response to exposure to foreign proteins; the body may make excessive antibodies to a transplanted kidney and cause rejection

Arteriovenous fistula A connection between an artery and a vein, typically in the forearm, for hemodialysis patients

Atherosclerosis Buildup of cholesterol-laden material on the walls of blood vessels; associated with coronary artery disease and hypertension

Azathioprine An immunosuppressant drug used to prevent organ rejection

Biopsy A medical procedure to remove a small amount of tissue from an organ, such as the kidney, for diagnosis

Blood Urea Nitrogen (BUN) The end-product of protein metabolism in the liver which is excreted by the kidneys. Its level rises with kidney failure

Body Mass Index (BMI) A value derived from the mass and height of an individual, defined as body mass divided by the square of body height

CRP Test A C-Reactive Protein test detects inflammation, either from an acute event like an infection, or from chronic disease

Calcium A mineral needed for bone health. Its availability is diminished in renal failure because of vitamin D deficiency

Continuous Ambulatory Peritoneal Dialysis (CAPD) A type of dialysis requiring a semi permeable membrane called the peritoneal membrane and fluid called dialysate which is exchanged 4 to 5 times a day

Corticoid Steroids Anti-inflammatory drugs such as prednisone used to treat auto immune diseases

Chronic Cyclic Peritoneal Dialysis (CCPD) A computerized machine that performs exchanges to cleanse the blood of waste products while a patient sleeps

Chronic Glomerulonephritis A progressive loss of kidney function that may follow an infection and leads to chronic renal failure

Creatinine An important indicator of renal health because it is an easily measured byproduct of muscle metabolism that is excreted unchanged by the kidneys

Dialysate Fluid and solutes in a dialysis process that flow through the dialyzer, do not pass through the membrane, and are discarded along with removed toxic substances after leaving the dialyzer

Dialysis Any means of cleansing the blood of waste products in patients with kidney failure

Donor-specific Antibodies Antibodies that bind to donor HLA and can injure or cause rejection of a transplanted kidney

Edema Swelling in body tissues caused by retention of salt and water

Erythropoietin A kidney-manufactured hormone that tells bone marrow to make red blood cells

Focal Segmental Glomerulosclerosis A kidney disease associated with nephrotic syndrome that progresses to chronic renal failure

Fistula A blood vessel access created by attaching a vein to an artery in the arm, but occasionally in the leg, for hemodialysis

Gamma Globulin A substance made from human blood plasma. The plasma, processed from donated human blood, contains antibodies that protect the body against diseases

Glomerular Filtration Rate (GFR) A measure of the kidneys' ability to excrete waste products through filtration in the glomerulus

Glomerulus The first part of the nephron composed of capillaries that filter waste products out of the blood to be excreted by the kidneys

HLA Typing A way to test a transplant candidate's immune compatibility with a potential donor

Hereditary Nephritis A slowly progressive inherited kidney disease, sometimes associated with deafness, that leads to chronic kidney failure

Hypothalamus A portion of the brain containing a number of small nuclei with a variety of functions, including linking the nervous system to the endocrine system via the pituitary gland

Hyperparathyroidism A disorder in which the parathyroid glands in the neck produce too much parathyroid hormone (PTH)

Immunoglobulin A large, Y-shaped protein produced mainly by plasma cells that is used by the immune system to identify and neutralize pathogens such as bacteria and viruses

Leptin A hormone predominantly made by adipose cells that helps regulate energy balance by inhibiting hunger

Nephrotic Syndrome A way that certain specific kidney diseases may manifest themselves. It is defined as proteinuria of at least 3.5 grams of protein in 24 hours and high levels of lipids in the blood

Metabolic Balance An equilibrium between the intake of nutrients and their eventual loss through absorption or excretion

Parathyroid Hormone (PTH) A hormone made in the four parathyroid glands located under the thyroid gland that is essential for calcium and phosphorus metabolism; PTH level rises in kidney failure and leads to bone disease and atherosclerosis

Peritonitis Inflammation of the peritoneal membrane, seen when a patient performing peritoneal dialysis develops infection

Polycystic Kidney Disease A disorder passed down through families; characterized by many large cysts in the kidneys

Pulmonary Renal Syndrome A severe disease process, caused by several different diseases that attack both the lungs and the kidneys

Resistin A cysteine-rich adipose-derived peptide hormone that in humans is encoded by the RETN gene

Septic A septic infection, also known as sepsis, is an infection of the blood that leads to septic shock and organ failure in severe cases

Thymus Gland A specialized organ of the immune system comprised of two identically sized lobes, located behind the sternum (breastbone), but in front of the heart

Transplantation Replacing a nonfunctioning organ with a healthy one from another person

Uremic Syndrome Symptoms experienced when kidney function falls below 15%

Vitamin D A group of fat-soluble secosteroids responsible for increasing intestinal absorption of calcium, magnesium, and phosphate, and multiple other biological effects

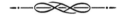

Glosario

Acidosis: Demasiado ácido en la sangre, directamente relacionado con la falla de los riñones para excretarlo.

Adenosina: Es una droga que se utiliza para que el corazón vuelva a su ritmo normal. También puede ser utilizada para realizar una prueba de corazón para la enfermedad de la arteria coronaria.

Adipocitos: Son células especializadas para el almacenamiento de grasa que se encuentran en el tejido conectivo.

Adiponectina: Es una hormona proteica que se encarga de regular los niveles de glucosa, así como la descomposición de los ácidos grasos.

Albúmina: Es una proteína que vive en el torrente sanguíneo y se concentra en el hígado. Cuando aparece en la orina es señal de enfermedad del riñón.

Anemia: Es un conteo bajo de glóbulos rojos con innumerables causas. Cuando falla el riñón para sintetizar eritropoyetina durante el curso de la insuficiencia renal, el paciente desarrolla anemia por insuficiencia renal.

Aneurisma: Es la debilidad en la pared de un gran vaso sanguíneo - frecuentemente causado por hipertensión - que conduce a un hinchamiento del vaso, que a su vez, puede romperse y llevar a la pérdida de sangre, potencialmente mortal.

Angiotensina 2: Es un poderoso agente que causa constricción severa de los vasos sanguíneos y subsecuentemente hipertensión. Cuando fallan los riñones, indirectamente, aumenta esta proteína.

Anticuerpo: Es una proteína sintetizada por el sistema inmune, en respuesta a la exposición a proteínas extrañas, el cuerpo puede crear anticuerpos excesivos a un riñón trasplantado y causar rechazo.

Anticuerpos específicos del donante: Son los anticuerpos que se unen a los antígenos leucocitarios humanos del donante (HLA) y pueden dañar o causar rechazo en un trasplante de riñón.

Anti-Diuretic Hormone (ADH): A protein stored and synthesized in the brain, released when a person is dehydrated. Kidneys respond to its release by retaining water and concentrating urine

Aterosclerosis: Es la acumulación de material cargado de colesterol en las paredes de los vasos sanguíneos asociado con la enfermedad de la arteria coronaria e hipertensión.

Azatioprina: Es una droga inmunosupresora utilizada para prevenir rechazo de órganos.

Balance Metabólico: Es un equilibrio entre la ingesta de nutrientes y la pérdida eventual por absorción o excreción.

Biopsia: Es un procedimiento médico para remover una pequeña cantidad de tejido de un órgano como el riñón, para un diagnóstico.

Calcio: Es un mineral necesario para la salud de los huesos. Su disponibilidad disminuye con la insuficiencia renal por la deficiencia de la vitamina D.

Creatinina: Es un indicador importante de la salud del riñón, porque es un subproducto que se mide fácilmente del metabolismo muscular que se excreta, sin consecuencias, por los riñones.

Diabetes en adultos: También llamada diabetes tipo 2. Es el resultado de un 95% de todos los casos de diabetes en el mundo y es la causa más común de insuficiencia renal.

Diálisis: Tiene que ver con la limpieza de la sangre de los productos de desecho en pacientes con deficiencia renal.

Diálisis peritoneal ambulatoria continua (CAPD): Es un tipo de diálisis que requiere una membrana semipermeable llamada membrana peritoneal y un fluido llamado dializado que se intercambia de 4 a 5 veces al día.

Diálisis peritoneal cíclica crónica (CCPD): Es una máquina computarizada que realiza cambios para limpiar la sangre de productos de desecho, mientras el paciente duerme.

Dializado: Es el fluido y solutos en un proceso de diálisis que fluye a través del dializador, no pasa a través de la membrana y se descargan junto con las sustancias tóxicas eliminadas después de salir del dializador.

Edema: Es la hinchazón en los tejidos del cuerpo, causada por la retención de sal y agua.

Enfermedad renal poliquística: Es un trastorno transmitido a través de las familias, caracterizado por muchos quistes grandes en los riñones.

Eritropoyetina: Es una hormona fabricada por el riñón que le indica a la médula ósea que produzca glóbulos rojos.

Esteroides Corticoides: Es una droga antiinflamatoria como la prednisona, utilizada para tratar enfermedades autoinmunes.

Fístula: Es un acceso a un vaso sanguíneo, creado al conectar una vena a una arteria en el brazo, pero, ocasionalmente, en la pierna para la hemodiálisis

Fístula Arteriovenosa: Es una conexión entre una arteria y una vena, típicamente en el antebrazo para pacientes en hemodiálisis.

Gama globulina: Es una sustancia hecha de plasma sanguíneo humano. El plasma, procesado de la sangre humana donada, contiene anticuerpos que protegen el cuerpo contra las enfermedades.

Glándula Timo: Es un órgano especializado del sistema inmunológico compuesto de lóbulos de tamaño idéntico, localizada detrás del esternón (quilla), frente al corazón.

Glándulas suprarrenales: Son pequeños órganos que se localizan en la parte superior de cada riñón, que secretan entre otras hormonas, aldosterona que causa que el riñón retenga sal y agua.

Glomérulo: Es una parte de la nefrona compuesta de capilares que filtran productos de desecho fuera de la sangre para ser excretados por los riñones.

Glomeruloesclerosis Segmentaria Focal: Es una enfermedad del riñón asociada con el síndrome nefrótico que supera a la insuficiencia renal crónica.

Glomerulonefritis crónica: Es una pérdida progresiva del funcionamiento del riñón que puede generar una infección y conducir a una insuficiencia renal crónica.

Hiperparatiroidismo: Es un desorden en el cual las glándulas paratiroides del cuello producen demasiadas hormonas paratiroideas (PTH).

Hipotálamo: Es una parte del cerebro que contiene un número de pequeños núcleos con una variedad de funciones, incluyendo la unión del sistema nervioso con el sistema endocrino a través de la glándula pituitaria.

Hormona Antidiurética (ADH): Es una proteína almacenada y sintetizada en el cerebro que se libera cuando una persona está deshidratada. Los riñones responden a su liberación al retener agua y concentrando la orina.

Índice de Masa Corporal: Es un valor derivado de la masa y peso de un individuo, se define como masa corporal, dividido por la altura del cuerpo.

Inmunoglobulina: Una gran proteína en forma de Y, producida principalmente por células de plasma que son utilizadas por el sistema inmunológico para identificar y neutralizar patógenos tales como bacterias y virus.

La Hormona Paratiroidea (PTH): Es una hormona producida en las cuatro glándulas paratiroides, localizadas debajo de la glándula tiroides que es esencial para el metabolismo del calcio y el fósforo. Los niveles de la PTH aumentan con la insuficiencia renal y conduce a la enfermedad ósea y aterosclerosis.

Leptina: Es una hormona predominantemente compuesta por células adiposas que ayudan a regular el balance de la energía, al inhibir el hambre.

Nefritis Hereditaria: Es una enfermedad renal hereditaria lentamente progresiva, algunas veces, asociada con sordera que conduce a una deficiencia de riñón crónica.

Nitrógeno Ureico en sangre (BUN): Es el producto final del metabolismo proteico en el hígado, el cual es excretado a través de los riñones. Su nivel aumenta con la insuficiencia renal.

Peritonitis: Es la inflamación de la membrana peritoneal, se ve cuando un paciente que realiza diálisis peritoneal, desarrolla una infección.

Prueba de ANA: Es una prueba de anticuerpos antinucleares que mide la cantidad y el patrón de anticuerpos en la sangre que trabaja contra el propio cuerpo (reacción autoinmune)

Prueba PCR o Análisis de Proteína C reactiva de alta sensibilidad (CRP Test): Detecta inflamación, ya sea por un evento agudo como una infección o por una enfermedad crónica.

Resistina: Es una hormona peptídica derivada de la adiposidad, rica en cisteína que en los humanos está codificado por el gene RETN.

Séptica: Es una infección séptica, también conocida como sepsis, es una infección de la sangre que conduce a un choque séptico y la falla de los órganos en casos severos.

Síndrome Nefrótico: Una forma en que ciertas enfermedades renales específicas se pueden manifestar. Se define como proteinuria de al menos 3.5 gramos de proteína en 24 horas y altos niveles de lípidos en la sangre.

Síndrome Renal Pulmonar: Un proceso de enfermedad severa causada por diferentes enfermedades que atacan a ambos pulmones y a los riñones.

Síndrome Urémico: Síntomas experimentados cuando la función renal cae debajo del 15%.

Tasa de Filtración Glomerular (GFR): Es una medida de la capacidad del riñón para excretar productos de desecho, a través de la filtración en el glomérulo.

Tipificación del HLA: Es una manera de probar la compatibilidad inmune con un donador potencial para un trasplante.

Trasplante: Es el reemplazo de un órgano que no funciona, por uno sano de otra persona.

Vitamina D: Es un grupo de secosteroides solubles en grasa, responsables del aumento de la absorción intestinal del calcio, magnesio y fosfato y de otros múltiples efectos biológicos.

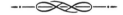

About the Author

Dr. Michael Barry Fisher, son of an educator/coach and housewife, was born in Brooklyn, where he spent his first 25 years. A natural athlete, he dreamed of being a professional pitcher until future Red Sox star Rico Petrocelli hit a ball off him that still hasn't landed.

At a young age, he read A. J. Cronin's The Citadel, a 1937 novel about medical injustice, malpractice and insensitivity in the coal-mining towns of South Wales. In his middle-school yearbook, he called it his favorite book, and listed "doctor" as his future profession. Prescient, indeed.

In high school, Dr. Fisher learned about Project Hope and its hospital ship, the SS Hope. He was drawn to the combination of far-flung adventure and providing medical care to underserved third-world countries. Though he never travelled on that ship, these notions nourished a taproot that would grow to feed the branches of his personal and professional life.

At the State University of New York Upstate Medical University, Dr. Fisher gravitated to internal medicine because it required physiological knowledge of each organ system and challenged doctors to be detectives, diagnosticians, and problem-solvers. Maybe most important, it required doctor/patient relationships, central to his worldview and future career.

In a pathology course, his professor had a special interest in the kidney, and was one of the first to study a glomerulus under an electron microscope. During class, lights would blink off and spectacular electron micrographs of the glomerulus would appear on a big screen. His curiosity piqued, he wanted to know more about this fascinating organ. In his senior year, he read Harrison's Textbook of Medicine and found himself drawn still further to kidneys, their function and dysfunction. During his oral final exam in Internal Medicine, his examiner turned out to be a nephrologist who asked questions about nephrotic syndrome, glomerulonephritis, and metabolic acidosis.

Not surprisingly, he got an "A."

During that senior year of med school, Lady Luck tapped his shoulder. Her name was Leslie Schiller, a Master's student in education at Syracuse University whom he found engaging, unpretentious and beautiful. They fell in love and married in December 1968. Forty-seven years later, she remains his best friend, confidant, moral compass, and mother to three wonderful children.

Leslie had been accepted into the Peace Corps but chose to delay entering the program until after she got her Master's degree. It was a complex time in American history. The Vietnam War raged abroad, protests raged at home. Leslie and Dr. Fisher decided to join the Peace Corps together, to serve their country while enjoying the adventure of living in a third-world nation and contributing to international cooperation—a modified version of his childhood dream, a terrestrial version of the Hope Ship.

They were assigned to La Paz, Bolivia, in the Andes, 13,000 feet above sea level. Dr. Fisher served as staff physician for Peace Corps volunteers. Leslie taught in a girl's reform school. He also established outpatient clinics and rumbled by jeep to villages in the Altiplano, conducting clinics for the Aymara indigenous people. He once treated a boy with nephrotic syndrome, whose father paid him with a chicken and basket of eggs—far more than he ever expected, more humbling as well.

After two years in South America, Dr. Fisher and Leslie returned stateside, where he completed his medical residency and two years of renal fellowship at UCLA. Then they discovered Santa Barbara and fell in love again, this time with beautiful city 100 miles north of Los Angeles, bordered by mountains and ocean, where they've remained ever since.

During that time, and throughout Dr. Fisher's practice, from Bolivia to UCLA to Santa Barbara, the notion of hope has guided the human side of his medical approach, a lodestone for treating patients with "high tech and high touch."

Grounding his practice in the notion of hope, he says, has given his life a sense of purpose. It's part of the human spirit that can never be defeated, and an aspect of medicine critical to curing the chronically ill. Case histories in this book help demonstrate that hope, combined with sound medical care, courage, and resilience, can carry the day in the face of seemingly insurmountable odds.

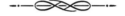

Made in the USA
San Bernardino, CA
11 June 2018